Soner Şahin and Kenan Demir
Editors

Bioprinting the Human

Medicine & Health
New York

DOI: https://doi.org/10.52305/PYRA1955.

NOTICE TO THE READER

Additional color graphics may be available in the e-book version of this book.

Library of Congress Cataloging-in-Publication Data

ISBN: 978-1-68507-993-2

Published by Nova Science Publishers, Inc. † New York

New Developments in Medical Research

Evidence-Based Medicine:
From the Clinician and Educator Perspective
Sowdhamini Wallace, DO, MS (Editor)
Ganga Gokulakrishnan, MD, MS (Editor)
2022. ISBN: 978-1-68507-546-0 (Hardcover)
2022. ISBN: 978-1-68507-700-6 (eBook)

COVID-19 by Cases: A Pandemic Review
Sujanthy S. Rajaram, MD, MPH, FACP, FAASM, FCCM (Editor)
Anthony Longo, MD (Editor)
Nicole Burak, MD (Editor)
2021. ISBN: 978-1-68507-099-1 (Hardcover)
2021. ISBN: 978-1-68507-262-9 (eBook)

Respiratory Care in Non Invasive Mechanical
Ventilatory Support: Principles and Practice
Antonio M. Esquinas, M.D, PhD (Editor)
Mohammed Alahmari, PhD (Editor)
2021. ISBN: 978-1-53619-702-0 (Hardcover)
2021. ISBN: 978-1-53619-902-4 (eBook)

Platelet-Rich Plasma:
Myths vs. Reality, Health Effects, and Risks
Pietro Gentile, MD, PhD
2021. ISBN: 978-1-53619-722-8 (eBook)

An Occupational Therapist's Role
in Health Literacy and Integrated Care
Brittany Ferri, PhD, OTR/L, CPRP
2021 ISBN: 978-1-53619-549-1 (Hardcover)
2021 ISBN: 978-1-53619-679-5 (eBook)

More information about this series can be found at
https://novapublishers.com/product-category/series/new-developments-in-medical-research/

New Developments in Medical Research

nova
Medicine & Health
New York

Contents

Preface

Rapidly developing technology also gives direction to our lives in the field of health and medicine. New developments are taking both diagnosis and treatment possibilities to places we could not predict before. The development of tissues and organs in a laboratory environment is one of these developments. This issue, which came to the fore with the introduction of 3D printers into our lives, has now started to mature and experiment in the field of medicine. Using a technology similar to 3D printing that fundamentally changes therapeutic possibilities, bioprinting uses a digital file as a blueprint to produce biomedical parts that closely mimic the properties of natural tissue. Engineered textures are created by layering biomaterials and/or living cells, collectively called bioinks. Transplanting the tissues or organs obtained to the needy patient also prevents possible undesirable situations such as tissue and organ rejection. This book on bioprinting aims to present the basics of bioprinting and its use in major tissues to the reader with the latest developments.

Acknowledgments

As the editors, we would like to thank Nişantaşı University for their support.

Chapter 1

What is Bioprinting?

Fatmagül İlayda Aydınlı[1] and Muhammet Volkan Bülbül[2,*]

[1]Department of Medical Biology,
School of Medicine, Nisantasi University,
Istanbul, Turkey
[2]Department of Histology and Embryology,
School of Medicine, Nisantasi University,
Istanbul, Turkey

Abstract

3D bioprinting reprocesses medical imaging data to produce complex tissues and organs using bioinks consisting of cells, biomaterials, and growth factors. Bioprinting holds realistic shapes and sizes of tissue and organs without losing any functionality. Due to the limited number of donors and immune rejection, studies of tissue and organ fabrication with 3D bioprinting have become the focus area of regenerative medicine and tissue engineering. 3D bioprinting uses various techniques such as inkjet-based bioprinting, laser-assisted bioprinting, and extrusion-based bioprinting to perform drug testing and delivery analysis, in addition to tissue and organ fabrication, and tissue engineering research. Although there are still certain challenges and limitations of 3D bioprinting processes, it is promising that with the increase in the number of future studies and technological developments, the printing of functional human organs and transplantations will become reality. Most importantly, it is strongly believed that 3D bioprinting can overcome the whole organ

* Corresponding Author's Email: volkan.bulbul@nisantasi.edu.tr.

In: Bioprinting the Human
Editors: Soner Şahin and Kenan Demir
ISBN: 978-1-68507-993-2

transplantation problem, which will revolutionize the field of the healthcare industry.

Keywords: 3D bioprinting, tissue engineering, bioinks, bioprinting

Introduction

The main limiting reason for organ transplantations is the low number of donors. Furthermore, the functionality of donated organs and the risk of disease or infection arising from individuals cause a significant reduction in the number of healthy tissues available (Neuberger & Callaghan, 2020; Shah et al., 2020). With the Covid-19 pandemic that all people around the world have been exposed to recently, these limiting factors have become more vital. A small organ pool can be created with organs obtained from living donors. Since current demand cannot be met, many people die while waiting for a transplant (Girlanda, 2016). For this reason, research on the development of alternative methods to obtain functional tissues is actively continuing (Cui et al., 2017a). In response to high demand, the use of three-dimensional (3D) printing technology in tissue engineering research and medical applications has made massive progress in recent years (Y. S. Zhang et al., 2018).

In 3D printing, with the help of computer-aided design (CAD) and segmentation software, 3D models' files are created using two-dimensional (2D) medical images and then physically printed (Ali et al., 2018; Mitsouras et al., 2015). Many branches of medicine use 3D printing technology for surgical procedures, educational processes, and implantable medical device production. In 3D printing processes, non-biological cell-free materials, such as gel and powder, are used in the production of the material to be created (Ravnic et al., 2017; Vijayavenkataraman et al., 2018).

Recently, "bioprinting" has emerged as a new process that is heard in studies by researchers in this field. In bioprinting processes, unlike conventional 3D printing, solutions containing biological materials and cells mixed with growth factors, or cells alone, are used to create the material (Ravnic et al., 2017). One of the main issues in 3D bioprinting of human tissues is the formulation of bioinks to be used (J. Zhang et al., 2021). When the components are created, their printability, strength, and biocompatibility must be tested. In addition, attention should be paid to factors such as proper adhesion of cells, immune response, biodegradability, mechanical properties, and structural integrity (O'Brien, 2011; Y.S. Zhang et al., 2018). Layer-by-layer construction of tissue can be produced with high precision, repeatability, and reproducibility thanks to 3D bioprinting (Kačarević et al., 2018; Li et al., 2016). To mimic the real situation, in particular homeostasis, 3D bioprinting technology retains the ability to control the cellular orientation of tissues, the external shape, and the internal geometry of a cell (Lee & Yeong, 2016; Murphy et al., 2020). With the right selection of bioinks used in 3D bioprinting, tissue integrity can be achieved by controlled releases of growth factors and bioactive substances (Gungor-Ozkerim et al., 2018; Y. S. Zhang et al., 2017; Zhu et al., 2016). In these aspects, 3D bioprinting provides advantages over scaffold-based modeling and printing, which is considered a relatively old method (Y. S. Zhang et al., 2017).

Organ transplantation, drug test analysis, realistic imitation of natural tissues, and printing are among the studies of 3D bioprinting. For this reason, it is strongly promising for studies on the development of new tissue and organ models. Today, many 3D bioprinting methods are applied and improved for the production of various tissue architectures, such as extrusion bioprinting, inkjet bioprinting, laser-assisted bioprinting, and light-mediated stereolithography (Derakhshanfar et al., 2018; Mandrycky et al., 2016). Most importantly, 3D bioprinting applications provide a multidisciplinary working platform by bringing together the fields of developmental biology, cell biology, regenerative medicine, bioengineering, and especially tissue engineering (Bishop et al., 2017).

Bioprinting Process

The 3D bioprinting process carried out with the coordination of different disciplines includes three important issues: the proper selection and preparation of the materials used in bioprinting, the actual printing process, and finally the post-production stabilization of the bioprinted model.

The first step is considered as the (1) preparation. The digital 3D models to be printed are prepared from 2D files at this point. Also, the determination of the right cell types and materials is another important issue of this step. In the (2) processing step, the actual bioprinting process occurs with the proper printing method. At the post-processing step (3), experiments are carried out that control the stabilization of the bioprinted 3D model (Bishop et al., 2017; Matai et al., 2020) (Figure 1).

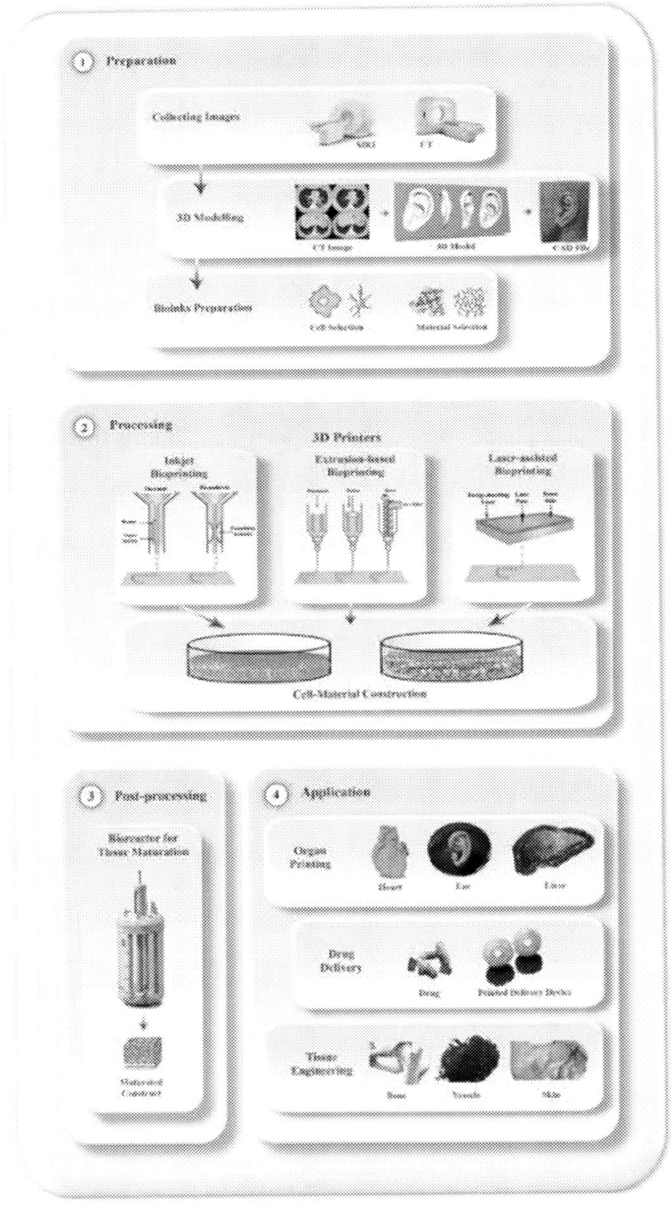

Figure 1. Process and application of 3D bioprinting. Inspired by Jin et al., 2021; Maina et al., 2018; Pasparakis et al., 2010; Saini et al., 2021.

Preparation

To proceed with the preparation step properly, it is necessary to understand the basic anatomical characteristics of the tissue. The selection of the imaging method is largely dependent on the characteristics of the tissue and determines the resolution and accuracy of the 3D model to be created. In this step, 2D images obtained through technologies such as computed tomography (CT) or magnetic resonance imaging (MRI) scans are reconstructed to design 3D models (Xing et al., 2020). 3D bioprinting processes were developed using traditional 3D printing methods. Models designed in CAD software are converted to an STL (standard tessellation language) file to represent objects in a three-dimensional Cartesian coordinate system bioprinter (Mohan Pandey et al., 2003). Relevant information on the color, texture, and surface geometry of objects is loaded specifically into the 3D bioprinting. Afterward, the model to be used by the printer and the appropriate printing material are selected. Most importantly, the necessary cell types and materials are selected for the procedure (Xing et al., 2020). Since this is an essential step, it will be discussed in detail in the bioinks section.

Bioinks

The materials used for 3D bioprinting are defined as bioinks. Cells, materials, and supporting factors are essential components of bioinks that play a significant role in the manufacturing of living artificial tissues and organs (Jamieson et al., 2021). Bioinks are inks known for their printability and cell compatibility. Although their printability capabilities are important for the fidelity of the shape and mechanical stability of the printed model, their cytocompatibility determines cell viability, proliferation, differentiation, and subsequent tissue formation. Since there are many parameters to consider, the selection of bioinks should be made according to the type of bioprinter and the tissue to be printed.

Biomaterials act as reinforcers for growing cells by supporting adhesion, proliferation, and functionality (O'Brien, 2011; Y. S. Zhang et al., 2018). Biomaterials used in tissue engineering are divided into three groups: natural polymers, synthetic polymers, and ceramics (O'Brien, 2011). Natural polymers include components of the extracellular matrix such as collagen, fibrin, proteoglycans, and biological materials found naturally in the body (Augustine, 2018). They are widely used in bioprinting due to their high biological activity and compatibility with cells and their microenvironment (Xing et al., 2020). Synthetic polymers include chemically synthesized compounds such as polystyrene, polylactic acid, and polyethylene glycol. Although synthetic polymers cannot provide an extracellular matrix with the same efficiency as natural polymers, they can specifically meet the needs of particular tissue structures (O'Brien, 2011; Y. S. Zhang et al., 2018). Due to these characteristics, the physical and chemical properties of bioinks can be easily manipulated and controlled (Xing et al., 2020). Ceramics are not as widely used as natural or synthetic polymers. However, they participate in the formation of 3D models of hard tissue structures such as bone (Diloksumpan et al., 2020). Ceramics consist of minerals such as calcium, phosphates, and hydroxyapatites, which are abundant in the bone tissue matrix. Additionally, ceramic-based scaffolds interact positively with osteocytes to develop the stiffness of the tissue.

In addition to biomaterials, the choice of the right cell line is also important in the process. It plays a crucial role in determining the design and functionality of the constructed tissue (Polak & Mantalaris, 2008). Many factors are considered when selecting a cell line, including cell source, number of cells, cell viability, and intended function (Augustine, 2018). But also, compatibility with biomaterials is essential for the integrity and functionality of the tissue constructed. Somatic cells such as chondrocytes, fibroblasts, and cardiac myocytes are often used in 3D bioprinting (Albanna et al., 2019; Martínez Ávila et al., 2016). However, in most applications, stem cells are also included in the formulation to facilitate de novo tissue development. In this way, their differentiation, unlimited cell proliferation, and high regeneration capabilities are utilized in the 3D bioprinting process (Ong et al., 2018).

Processing

Bioinks containing the cell line and biomaterials, the 3D scaffold printing method, and various additive manufacturing techniques were determined in the previous step. In the production of the processing step, the physical 3D model of tissues or organs is carried out (Bishop et al., 2017; Bose et al., 2013). Inkjet-based, laser-assisted, and extrusion-based bioprinting is popularly preferred for this production.

Inkjet Bioprinting

Inspired by desktop printers, inkjet bioprinting has been redesigned to print living cells on 3D structures using special bioinks and it was the first bioprinting technology used in this field (Tuan et al., 2003). Inkjet bioprinting has a function of non-contact printing in which liquid bioinks are loaded into the nozzle and the droplets are carefully placed on the surface of the constructed tissue (Augustine, 2018). With this method, multiple cells or proteins are placed in a targeted spatial position with more than one print head, allowing the production of complex multicellular structures (Ker et al., 2011; Li et al., 2016; Xu et al., 2009). Compared to other 3D bioprinting techniques, inkjet bioprinting has advantages in terms of speed, high output capacity, high resolution, low cost, high cell viability, and reproducibility (Roth et al., 2004).

Laser-Assisted Bioprinting

Bioprinting using laser sources is the advanced conversion technique for transferring biological material such as peptides, DNA, and cells to 3D models (Colina et al., 2005; Ringeisen et al., 2004). In the laser-assisted bioprinting process, there is no direct contact between the bioinks and the disperser, therefore this situation provides cell protection from being stressed, resulting in high cell viability (Mandrycky et al., 2016). Also, they do not use a nozzle for the delivery of bioinks. Laser-assisted bioprinting creates 3D structures using pulsed or continuous monochromatic laser energy, and consequently, it offers high resolution, high cell viability, high cell density, and rapid production. However, it has disadvantages due to the higher maintenance costs compared to other types of production and the potential to cause cell damage in the case of cells exposed to laser energy (Khoda et al., 2013; Vijayavenkataraman et al., 2018; Y. S. Zhang et al., 2018).

Extrusion-Based Bioprinting

Extrusion-based bioprinting is the most widely used by several researchers as a manufacturing technique where bioinks come out continuously from the nozzle and mechanical compressions or pneumatic pressure are used to create layered constructs (Fedorovich et al., 2010; Vijayavenkataraman et al., 2018; Wüst et al., 2014). In this technique, both the liquid delivery system and the automatic robotic system are combined for extrusion and printing (Mironov et al., 2003). Due to the wide range of bioink viscosities used, extrusion-based bioprinting is preferred for creating large and stable 3D tissue constructs. Another reason for the preference is that the consistency of bioinks used in the extrusion technique tends to coalesce into pastes or dispersions with higher viscosity compared to other methods (Tan et al., 2021). One of the advantages of extrusion-based bioprinters is their ability to print a wide range of biomaterials such as cell spheroids, hydrogels, and biocompatible copolymers (Jones, 2012). In addition, they have low production costs and high-density cell capacity (Vijayavenkataraman et al., 2018). The most important disadvantage of extrusion-based bioprinting is that it has a very low resolution at around 100 μm (Duan et al., 2013). Additionally, disadvantages include slower production times, an increased risk of clogging the extrusion nozzle with bioinks, and reduced cell viability during bioprinting (Murphy & Atala, 2014).

Post-Processing

The post-processing phase includes studies in which 3D tissue constructs must be maintained in vitro for maturation before in vivo implantation (J. Zhang et al., 2021). These conditions are achieved in vitro using bioreactors in which the environment mimics natural tissue (Santoro et al., 2010). Supplying chemical, physical stimuli, and nutrients to bioreactors increase the differentiation and maturation of cells (Rosser & Thomas, 2018). Bioreactor systems can be diversified according to the intended function as static systems, perfusion bioreactors, and spinning/rotating vessels (Ahmed et al., 2019). In each of these systems, there are many types and special devices designed to mimic the physiological conditions that tissue constructs need.

Application of Bioprinting

In recent years, 3D bioprinting studies have been widely developed and 3D printed models have been used in various fields such as medicine, health, and food technology. The potential medical uses of 3D bioprinting can be examined in several categories: drug discovery, tissue or organ fabrication, and tissue engineering (Dodziuk, 2016; Gupta & Bit, 2021; Saini et al., 2021).

Furthermore, extensive studies are still required for the improvement and development of the field of bioprinting (Bejoy et al., 2021).

Tissue Engineering

3D bioprinted implantation of major body tissues such as bone, cartilage, blood vessels, and skin has been carried out successfully (Saini et al., 2021). Bone and cartilage are considered hard tissue consisting of specific cell types of osteoblast cells with calcified extracellular matrix and cartilage chondrocyte cells, respectively. The 3D bioprinting process of hard tissue constructs requires the biomaterials to provide solid mechanical support to these cell types (Sun et al., 2018). Since bone is a connective tissue composed of osteoblasts, osteocytes, osteoclasts, and the surrounding calcified extracellular matrix, the selected biomaterials must be biocompatible, printable, and most importantly support cell viability (J. Zhang et al., 2021). In terms of cartilage tissue production, promoting chondrogenesis in cartilage-based tissue engineering is essential for viability (Kundu et al., 2015). Today, a great deal of research states that materials containing alginate and methacrylate are blended with appropriate hydrogel and cartilage cells to support the chondrocyte phenotype.

In addition to hard tissues, the 3D bioprinting technique is also convenient for printing artificial soft tissue. However, producing soft tissue with 3D bioprinting is more problematic, and skin is one of them (Gupta & Bit, 2021). Many cell types and functional structures, such as blood vessels, are involved in the formation of the skin, resulting in its more complex structure. Despite these challenges, numerous 3D bioprinting experiments have been carried out to create skin texture and have successfully achieved skin healing and growth in vitro and in vivo (Hong et al., 2018). The lack of vascularization that supplies skin tissue with essential nutrients and oxygen restricts the proper function of 3D bioprinted skin constructs. To overcome these limitations, the integration of endothelial cell printing into skin tissue constructs may provide the vascular network to maintain viability (Koch et al., 2012).

Organ Printing

The general method for the treatment of increasing organ failure or dysfunction due to traumatic injury and disease is transplantation from a recently deceased or living volunteer donor (Cui et al., 2017b). Clinical treatments are limited due to the low number of donors and low immune compatibility rates of donated tissues. Recently, 3D organ bioprinting approaches have been investigated as a promising solution in the search for alternatives to traditional treatment strategies. Researchers continue to work on the development of functional, full-size organs using regenerative medicine technology, and the 3D bioprinting process has promising results within this field. Many studies demonstrate that the heart, bladder, ear, and cornea have been artificially produced by 3D bioprinting (Saini et al., 2021). Human organs are highly complex structures in which many types of tissue function in an organized manner; therefore, whole organ bioprinting has some obstacles due to the complexities (Y. S. Zhang et al., 2017). To address the challenges, some of the current research focuses on the fabrication of vascularized tissue and its functionalization to improve the 3D bioprinting of organ studies (Gao et al., 2018; Jin et al., 2021).

Drug Delivery

3D bioprinting applications are not limited to tissue production or transplantations; they can also be used for drug delivery in drug test analysis studies. In particular, using 3D bioprinting for drug delivery scaffolds encourages the studies of personalized disease treatment, which are relatively less explored areas (Dey & Ozbolat, 2020). The incorporation of 3D bioprinting systems into drug delivery studies provides a highly efficient methodology for evaluating implant integration, as well as pathological and toxicological conditions in vitro. Moreover, 3D biomimetic microfluidic chips used in drug delivery have great potential to replace animal studies (Kačarević et al., 2018). In this sense, it will also contribute to the elimination of ethical concerns and limitations and may encourage a significant reduction in the number of animal experiments in the future.

Conclusion

To overcome the problem of organ transplantation, the printing of functional human organs is one of the most important issues in the healthcare industry. Over the past few years, research on new techniques and strategies to advance 3D bioprinting technology has been accelerated for this purpose. In addition, the 3D bioprinting process demonstrated that tissue can be regenerated, wound areas can be repaired, and all functional artificial tissues such as bone, skin, vessels, and heart can be created with cell-loaded scaffolds thanks to the combination of novel stem cell technologies and engineering. By presenting many examples of different 3D bioprinting technologies, researchers demonstrate the potential for tissue engineering to improve with this technology. Future studies of 3D bioprinting will dominate the field of tissue regeneration, allowing the fabrication of more complex tissue structures and medical applications. 3D bioprinting-based approaches to study drug delivery can be adopted in the pharmaceutical industry.

However, there are still certain problems and limitations encountered in 3D bioprinting processes. 3D bioprinted organs or tissues based on 2D imaging data may be affected by imaging errors. Therefore, accurate imaging of patient-specific tissues or organs is required to create the exact same tissue. In addition, optimization of bioinks is another challenge of the 3D bioprinting process. Because bioinks are exposed to high pressure and frequency or heat generated from bioreactors, it is essential to create the appropriate cellular environment to meet the requirements of particular cells. Moreover, although many studies have been done within the field of tissue engineering, there are still some tissue- or organ-specific limitations that need to be exceeded in the production. Finally, regulations are needed on the patentability and accessibility of 3D bioprinting technology.

Consequently, the combination of imaging techniques, bioinks, and 3D bioprinting technologies will bring a new concept to tissue engineering and regenerative medicine. 3D bioprinting will be the most promising method in the manufacture of 3D cell-based constructs to repair injured areas of tissue.

References

Ahmed, S., Chauhan, V. M., Ghaemmaghami, A. M., & Aylott, J. W. (2019). New generation of bioreactors that advance extracellular matrix modelling and tissue engineering. *Biotechnology Letters*, *41*(1), 1–25. https://doi.org/10.1007/s10529-018-2611-7.

Albanna, M., Binder, K. W., Murphy, S. v., Kim, J., Qasem, S. A., Zhao, W., Tan, J., El-Amin, I. B., Dice, D. D., Marco, J., Green, J., Xu, T., Skardal, A., Holmes, J. H., Jackson, J. D., Atala, A., & Yoo, J. J. (2019). In situ bioprinting of autologous skin cells accelerates wound healing of extensive excisional full-thickness wounds. *Scientific Reports*, *9*(1), 1856. https://doi.org/10.1038/s41598-018-38366-w.

Ali, M., P.R., A. K., Lee, S. J., & Jackson, J. D. (2018). Three-dimensional bioprinting for organ bioengineering: promise and pitfalls. *Current Opinion in Organ Transplantation*, *23*(6), 649–656. https://doi.org/10.1097/MOT.0000000000000581.

Augustine, R. (2018). Skin bioprinting: a novel approach for creating artificial skin from synthetic and natural building blocks. *Progress in Biomaterials*, *7*(2), 77–92. https://doi.org/10.1007/s40204-018-0087-0.

Badylak, S. F., Weiss, D. J., Caplan, A., & Macchiarini, P. (2012). RETRACTED: Engineered whole organs and complex tissues. *The Lancet*, *379*(9819), 943–952. https://doi.org/10.1016/S0140-6736(12)60073-7.

Bejoy, A. M., Makkithaya, K. N., Hunakunti, B. B., Hegde, A., Krishnamurthy, K., Sarkar, A., Lobo, C. F., Keshav, D. V. S., G, D., S, D. D., Mascarenhas, S., Chakrabarti, S., Kalepu, S. R. R. D., Paul, B., & Mazumder, N. (2021). An insight on advances and applications of 3D bioprinting: A review. *Bioprinting*, *24*, e00176. https://doi.org/10.1016/j.bprint.2021.e00176.

Bishop, E. S., Mostafa, S., Pakvasa, M., Luu, H. H., Lee, M. J., Wolf, J. M., Ameer, G. A., He, T.-C., & Reid, R. R. (2017). 3-D bioprinting technologies in tissue engineering and regenerative medicine: Current and future trends. *Genes & Diseases*, *4*(4), 185–195. https://doi.org/10.1016/j.gendis.2017.10.002.

Bose, S., Vahabzadeh, S., & Bandyopadhyay, A. (2013). Bone tissue engineering using 3D printing. *Materials Today*, *16*(12), 496–504. https://doi.org/10.1016/j.mattod. 2013.11.017.

Colina, M., Serra, P., Fernández-Pradas, J. M., Sevilla, L., & Morenza, J. L. (2005). DNA deposition through laser induced forward transfer. *Biosensors and Bioelectronics*, *20*(8), 1638–1642. https://doi.org/10.1016/j.bios.2004.08.047.

Cui, H., Nowicki, M., Fisher, J. P., & Zhang, L. G. (2017a). 3D Bioprinting for organ regeneration. *Advanced Healthcare Materials*, *6*(1). https://doi.org/10.1002/adhm.201601118.

Derakhshanfar, S., Mbeleck, R., Xu, K., Zhang, X., Zhong, W., & Xing, M. (2018). 3D bioprinting for biomedical devices and tissue engineering: A review of recent trends and advances. *Bioactive Materials*, *3*(2), 144–156. https://doi.org/10.1016/j.bioactmat.2017.11.008.

Dey, M., & Ozbolat, I. T. (2020). 3D bioprinting of cells, tissues and organs. *Scientific Reports*, *10*(1), 14023. https://doi.org/10.1038/s41598-020-70086-y.

Diloksumpan, P., de Ruijter, M., Castilho, M., Gbureck, U., Vermonden, T., van Weeren, P. R., Malda, J., & Levato, R. (2020). Combining multi-scale 3D printing technologies to engineer reinforced hydrogel-ceramic interfaces. *Biofabrication*, *12*(2), 025014. https://doi.org/10.1088/1758-5090/ab69d9.

Dodziuk, H. (2016). Applications of 3D printing in healthcare. *Polish Journal of Cardio-Thoracic Surgery*, *3*, 283–293. https://doi.org/10.5114/kitp.2016.62625.

Duan, B., Hockaday, L. A., Kang, K. H., & Butcher, J. T. (2013). 3D bioprinting of heterogeneous aortic valve conduits with alginate/gelatin hydrogels. *Journal of Biomedical Materials Research. Part A*, *101*(5), 1255–1264. https://doi.org/10.1002/jbm.a.34420.

Fedorovich, N. E., Haverslag, R. T., Dhert, W. J. A., & Alblas, J. (2010). The role of endothelial progenitor cells in prevascularized bone tissue engineering: development of heterogeneous constructs. *Tissue Engineering Part A*, *16*(7), 2355–2367. https://doi.org/10.1089/ten.tea.2009.0603.

Gao, G., Huang, Y., Schilling, A. F., Hubbell, K., & Cui, X. (2018). Organ bioprinting: are we there yet? *Advanced Healthcare Materials*, *7*(1), 1701018. https://doi.org/10.1002/adhm.201701018.

Girlanda, R. (2016). Deceased organ donation for transplantation: Challenges and opportunities. *World Journal of Transplantation*, *6*(3), 451–459. https://doi.org/10.5500/wjt.v6.i3.451.

Gungor-Ozkerim, P. S., Inci, I., Zhang, Y. S., Khademhosseini, A., & Dokmeci, M. R. (2018). Bioinks for 3D bioprinting: an overview. *Biomaterials Science*, *6*(5), 915–946. https://doi.org/10.1039/C7BM00765E.

Gupta, S., & Bit, A. (2021). 3D bioprinting in tissue engineering and regenerative medicine. *Cell and Tissue Banking*. https://doi.org/10.1007/s10561-021-09936-6.

Hong, N., Yang, G. H., Lee, J. H., & Kim, G. H. (2018). 3D bioprinting and its in vivo applications. In *Journal of Biomedical Materials Research - Part B Applied* - (Vol. 106, Issue 1, pp. 444–459). John Wiley and Sons Inc. https://doi.org/10.1002/jbm.b.33826.

Jamieson, C., Keenan, P., Kirkwood, D., Oji, S., Webster, C., Russell, K. A., & Koch, T. G. (2021). A review of recent advances in 3D bioprinting with an eye on future regenerative therapies in veterinary medicine. In *Frontiers in Veterinary Science* (Vol. 7). Frontiers Media S.A. https://doi.org/10.3389/fvets.2020.584193.

Jin, Z., Li, Y., Yu, K., Liu, L., Fu, J., Yao, X., Zhang, A., & He, Y. (2021). 3D printing of physical organ models: recent developments and challenges. *Advanced Science*, *8*(17), 2101394. https://doi.org/10.1002/advs.202101394.

Jones, N. (2012). Science in three dimensions: The print revolution. *Nature*, *487*(7405), 22–23. https://doi.org/10.1038/487022a.

Kačarević, Ž., Rider, P., Alkildani, S., Retnasingh, S., Smeets, R., Jung, O., Ivanišević, Z., & Barbeck, M. (2018). An introduction to 3D bioprinting: possibilities, challenges and future Aspects. *Materials*, *11*(11), 2199. https://doi.org/10.3390/ma11112199.

Ker, E. D. F., Chu, B., Phillippi, J. A., Gharaibeh, B., Huard, J., Weiss, L. E., & Campbell, P. G. (2011). Engineering spatial control of multiple differentiation fates within a stem cell population. *Biomaterials*, *32*(13), 3413–3422. https://doi.org/10.1016/ j.biomaterials.2011.01.036.

Khoda, A. K. M., Ozbolat, I. T., & Koc, B. (2013). Designing heterogeneous porous tissue scaffolds for additive manufacturing processes. *Computer-Aided Design*, *45*(12), 1507–1523. https://doi.org/10.1016/j.cad.2013.07.003.

Koch, L., Deiwick, A., Schlie, S., Michael, S., Gruene, M., Coger, V., Zychlinski, D., Schambach, A., Reimers, K., Vogt, P. M., & Chichkov, B. (2012). Skin tissue generation by laser cell printing. *Biotechnology and Bioengineering*, *109*(7), 1855–1863. https://doi.org/10.1002/bit.24455.

Kundu, J., Shim, J.-H., Jang, J., Kim, S.-W., & Cho, D.-W. (2015). An additive manufacturing-based PCL-alginate-chondrocyte bioprinted scaffold for cartilage tissue engineering. *Journal of Tissue Engineering and Regenerative Medicine*, *9*(11), 1286–1297. https://doi.org/10.1002/term.1682.

Lee, J. M., & Yeong, W. Y. (2016). Design and Printing Strategies in 3D Bioprinting of Cell-Hydrogels: A Review. *Advanced Healthcare Materials*, *5*(22), 2856–2865. https://doi.org/10.1002/adhm.201600435.

Li, J., Chen, M., Fan, X., & Zhou, H. (2016). Recent advances in bioprinting techniques: approaches, applications and future prospects. *Journal of Translational Medicine*, *14*(1), 271. https://doi.org/10.1186/s12967-016-1028-0.

Maina, R. M., Barahona, M. J., Finotti, M., Lysyy, T., Geibel, P., D'Amico, F., Mulligan, D., & Geibel, J. P. (2018). Generating vascular conduits: from tissue engineering to three-dimensional bioprinting. *Innovative Surgical Sciences*, *3*(3), 203–213. https://doi.org/10.1515/iss-2018-0016.

Mandrycky, C., Wang, Z., Kim, K., & Kim, D.-H. (2016). 3D bioprinting for engineering complex tissues. *Biotechnology Advances*, *34*(4), 422–434. https://doi.org/10.1016/j.biotechadv.2015.12.011.

Martínez Ávila, H., Schwarz, S., Rotter, N., & Gatenholm, P. (2016). 3D bioprinting of human chondrocyte-laden nanocellulose hydrogels for patient-specific auricular cartilage regeneration. *Bioprinting*, *1–2*, 22–35. https://doi.org/10.1016/j.bprint.2016.08.003.

Matai, I., Kaur, G., Seyedsalehi, A., McClinton, A., & Laurencin, C. T. (2020). Progress in 3D bioprinting technology for tissue/organ regenerative engineering. *Biomaterials*, *226*, 119536. https://doi.org/10.1016/j.biomaterials.2019.119536.

Mironov, V., Boland, T., Trusk, T., Forgacs, G., & Markwald, R. R. (2003). Organ printing: computer-aided jet-based 3D tissue engineering. *Trends in Biotechnology*, *21*(4), 157–161. https://doi.org/10.1016/S0167-7799(03)00033-7.

Mitsouras, D., Liacouras, P., Imanzadeh, A., Giannopoulos, A. A., Cai, T., Kumamaru, K. K., George, E., Wake, N., Caterson, E. J., Pomahac, B., Ho, V. B., Grant, G. T., & Rybicki, F. J. (2015). Medical 3D Printing for the Radiologist. *RadioGraphics*, *35*(7), 1965–1988. https://doi.org/10.1148/rg.2015140320.

Mohan Pandey, P., Venkata Reddy, N., & Dhande, S. G. (2003). Slicing procedures in layered manufacturing: a review. *Rapid Prototyping Journal*, *9*(5), 274–288. https://doi.org/10.1108/13552540310502185.

Murphy, S. v, & Atala, A. (2014). 3D bioprinting of tissues and organs. *Nature Biotechnology*, *32*(8), 773–785. https://doi.org/10.1038/nbt.2958.

Murphy, S. v., de Coppi, P., & Atala, A. (2020). Opportunities and challenges of translational 3D bioprinting. *Nature Biomedical Engineering*, *4*(4), 370–380. https://doi.org/10.1038/s41551-019-0471-7.

Neuberger, J., & Callaghan, C. (2020). Organ utilization – the next hurdle in transplantation? *Transplant International*, *33*(12), 1597–1609. https://doi.org/ 10.1111/tri.13744.

O'Brien, F. J. (2011). Biomaterials & scaffolds for tissue engineering. *Materials Today*, *14*(3), 88–95. https://doi.org/10.1016/S1369-7021(11)70058-X.

Ong, C. S., Yesantharao, P., Huang, C. Y., Mattson, G., Boktor, J., Fukunishi, T., Zhang, H., & Hibino, N. (2018). 3D bioprinting using stem cells. *Pediatric Research*, *83*(1–2), 223–231. https://doi.org/10.1038/pr.2017.252.

Pasparakis, G., Krasnogor, N., Cronin, L., Davis, B. G., & Alexander, C. (2010). Controlled polymer synthesis—from biomimicry towards synthetic biology. *Chem. Soc. Rev.*, *39*(1), 286–300. https://doi.org/10.1039/B809333B.

Polak, J. M., & Mantalaris, S. (2008). Stem cells bioprocessing: an important milestone to move regenerative medicine research into the clinical arena. *Pediatric Research*, *63*(5), 461–466. https://doi.org/10.1203/PDR.0b013e31816a8c1c.

Ravnic, D. J., Leberfinger, A. N., Koduru, S. v., Hospodiuk, M., Moncal, K. K., Datta, P., Dey, M., Rizk, E., & Ozbolat, I. T. (2017). Transplantation of bioprinted tissues and organs. *Annals of Surgery*, *266*(1), 48–58. https://doi.org/10.1097/SLA.0000000000002141.

Ringeisen, B. R., Kim, H., Barron, J. A., Krizman, D. B., Chrisey, D. B., Jackman, S., Auyeung, R. Y. C., & Spargo, B. J. (2004). Laser printing of pluripotent embryonal carcinoma cells. *Tissue Engineering*, *10*(3–4), 483–491. https://doi.org/ 10.1089/107632704323061843.

Rosser, J., & Thomas, D. J. (2018). Bioreactor processes for maturation of 3D bioprinted tissue. In *3D Bioprinting for Reconstructive Surgery* (pp. 191–215). Elsevier. https://doi.org/10.1016/B978-0-08-101103-4.00010-7.

Roth, E. A., Xu, T., Das, M., Gregory, C., Hickman, J. J., & Boland, T. (2004). Inkjet printing for high-throughput cell patterning. *Biomaterials*, *25*(17), 3707–3715. https://doi.org/10.1016/j.biomaterials.2003.10.052.

Saini, G., Segaran, N., Mayer, J. L., Saini, A., Albadawi, H., & Oklu, R. (2021). Applications of 3d bioprinting in tissue engineering and regenerative medicine. In *Journal of Clinical Medicine* (Vol. 10, Issue 21). MDPI. https://doi.org/10.3390/jcm10214966.

Santoro, R., Olivares, A. L., Brans, G., Wirz, D., Longinotti, C., Lacroix, D., Martin, I., & Wendt, D. (2010). Bioreactor based engineering of large-scale human cartilage grafts for joint resurfacing. *Biomaterials*, *31*(34), 8946–8952. https://doi.org/10.1016/j.biomaterials.2010.08.009.

Shah, M. B., Lynch, R. J., El-Haddad, H., Doby, B., Brockmeier, D., & Goldberg, D. S. (2020). Utilization of deceased donors during a pandemic: argument against using SARS-CoV-2–positive donors. *American Journal of Transplantation*, *20*(7), 1795–1799. https://doi.org/10.1111/ajt.15969.

Sun, T., Yao, S., Liu, M., Yang, Y., Ji, Y., Cui, W., Qu, Y., & Guo, X. (2018). Composite scaffolds of mineralized natural extracellular matrix on true bone ceramic induce bone regeneration through Smad1/5/8 and ERK1/2 pathways. *Tissue Engineering Part A*, *24*(5–6), 502–515. https://doi.org/10.1089/ten.tea.2017.0179.

Tan, B., Gan, S., Wang, X., Liu, W., & Li, X. (2021). Applications of 3D bioprinting in tissue engineering: advantages, deficiencies, improvements, and future perspectives. *Journal of Materials Chemistry B*, *9*(27), 5385–5413. https://doi.org/10.1039/D1TB00172H.

Tuan, R. S., Boland, G., & Tuli, R. (2003). Adult mesenchymal stem cells and cell-based tissue engineering. *Arthritis Research & Therapy*, *5*(1), 32. https://doi.org/10.1186/ar614.

Vijayavenkataraman, S., Yan, W.-C., Lu, W. F., Wang, C.-H., & Fuh, J. Y. H. (2018). 3D bioprinting of tissues and organs for regenerative medicine. *Advanced Drug Delivery Reviews, 132*, 296–332. https://doi.org/10.1016/j.addr.2018.07.004.

Wüst, S., Godla, M. E., Müller, R., & Hofmann, S. (2014). Tunable hydrogel composite with two-step processing in combination with innovative hardware upgrade for cell-based three-dimensional bioprinting. *Acta Biomaterialia, 10*(2), 630–640. https://doi.org/10.1016/j.actbio.2013.10.016.

Xing, F., Xiang, Z., Rommens, P. M., & Ritz, U. (2020). 3D Bioprinting for vascularized tissue-engineered bone fabrication. *Materials, 13*(10), 2278. https://doi.org/10.3390/ma13102278.

Xu, T., Baicu, C., Aho, M., Zile, M., & Boland, T. (2009). Fabrication and characterization of bio-engineered cardiac pseudo tissues. *Biofabrication, 1*(3), 035001. https://doi.org/10.1088/1758-5082/1/3/035001.

Zhang, J., Wehrle, E., Rubert, M., & Müller, R. (2021). 3d bioprinting of human tissues: Biofabrication, bioinks and bioreactors. In *International Journal of Molecular Sciences* (Vol. 22, Issue 8). MDPI AG. https://doi.org/10.3390/ijms22083971.

Zhang, Y. S., Oklu, R., Dokmeci, M. R., & Khademhosseini, A. (2018). Three-dimensional bioprinting strategies for tissue engineering. *Cold Spring Harbor Perspectives in Medicine, 8*(2). https://doi.org/10.1101/cshperspect.a025718.

Zhang, Y. S., Yue, K., Aleman, J., Mollazadeh-Moghaddam, K., Bakht, S. M., Yang, J., Jia, W., Dell'Erba, V., Assawes, P., Shin, S. R., Dokmeci, M. R., Oklu, R., & Khademhosseini, A. (2017). 3D bioprinting for tissue and organ fabrication. *Annals of Biomedical Engineering, 45*(1), 148–163. https://doi.org/10.1007/s10439-016-1612-8.

Zhu, W., Ma, X., Gou, M., Mei, D., Zhang, K., & Chen, S. (2016). 3D printing of functional biomaterials for tissue engineering. *Current Opinion in Biotechnology, 40*, 103–112. https://doi.org/10.1016/j.copbio.2016.03.014.

Chapter 2

3D-Printable Materials for Tissue Engineering

Kerim Emre Öksüz*
Department of Metallurgical & Materials Engineering,
Sivas Cumhuriyet University, Sivas, Turkey

Abstract

Medical applications for three-dimensional (3D) printing are spreading briskly and are anticipated to reform healthcare. The current and potential medical applications of 3D printing technology can be organized into several broad categories, including fabricating porous scaffolds, orthoses devices for tissue engineering, regenerative medicine, anatomical models, and the creation of customized prosthetics, implants, and drug delivery systems. 3D printing technology applicability in treatment can offer many advantages, such as individualization and personalization of medical products, drugs, high structural complexity, medical devices, and cost-efficiency. However, before 3D printing can be routinely used for the regeneration of complex tissues (e.g., muscle, bone, cartilage, vessels, craniomaxillofacial hard tissues) and complicated organs with complex 3D microarchitecture (e.g., liver, lymphoid organs), diverse restrictions such as biomaterial design parameters with tunable mechanical properties, optimal structures, degradation/bioactivity properties must be addressed. This book chapter will describe the leading polymer-based biomaterials and recent technological breakthroughs for the top 3D printing methods. 3D-printable polymer-based biomaterials, hydrogels, and bioinks will be highlighted according to their

* Corresponding Author's Email: emre.oksuz@cumhuriyet.edu.tr.

In: Bioprinting the Human
Editors: Soner Şahin and Kenan Demir
ISBN: 978-1-68507-993-2

processability, printability, fundamental limitations, and properties such as degradation rate, biocompatibility, and mechanics.

Keywords: tissue engineering, bioprinting, hydrogels, 3D printed scaffolds, biomaterials, polymers, regenerative medicine, mechanical properties, additive manufacturing

Introduction

3D Printing of Biomaterials for Tissue Engineering

Tissue engineering is an interdisciplinary discipline that combines the designs and rudiments of engineering and life sciences to solve clinical problems. Tissue engineering offers a promising alternative to restore functional tissues such as bone, neural tissues, skin, kidneys, heart, etc. The most significant advantages of tissue engineering are its capacity to overcome the limitations of traditional methods of implant transplantation and organ transplantation (Koch et al., 2010; Sachlos et al., 2003). In this context, tissue engineering is the function of engineering principles in chemistry, cell biology, medicine, and material science in conjunction with a mixture of physicochemical and biochemical factors to reconstruct the function of injured or infected tissue. These physiochemical and biochemical factors are growth, cells, biomaterials, and extrinsic stimulants.

The capacity to design and produce complex three-dimensional biomaterials is an important area of biomedical engineering. Utilizations for 3D biomedical apparatus are the restoration of dental parts, 3D anatomic defects, prosthetic parts, craniofacial implants, reconstruction of complex organs with complicated 3D structure (such as thymus, bone marrow & liver), implantable biosensors, and scaffolds for tissue regeneration (Ahlfeld et al., 2021; Chu et al., 2021; Said et al., 2020; Yang et al., 2019). However, 3D printing has made considerable progress in producing patient-specific prostheses with high anatomical complicacy, organs for transplantation, and design flexibility. The continued advancement of 3D bioprinting technology (Figure 1) presents several challenges such as selection of biomaterials, tissue architecture and complexity, cell migration and viability, angiogenesis, and bioink properties (Kumar et al., 2019).

Additive manufacturing (commonly known as 3D printing) is a technology for the layer-by-layer manufacturing method of 3D objects.

Additive manufacturing uses computer-assisted design software (CAD) or a 3D object scanner to instruct the hardware to deposit the material layer by layer in precise geometric/complicated shapes. As is well-known, additive *manufacturing offers many advantages with developing technology. For example,* 3D printing enables the production of patient-specific 3D-printed implants, meaning an implant designed especially for a particular patient in terms of size and shape, and can be tailored to another patient's needs.

These custom-made implants can permanently replace injured tissue or strengthen tissue to encourage regeneration. In the latter case, a biodegradable scaffold can support the structure of the forming tissue. As a result of these factors, multiple additive manufacturing technologies for the 3D printing of diverse materials have arisen (Kolesky et al., 2014). According to ASTM standards, additive manufacturing technologies are branched into seven types, depending on the techniques used to produce these 3D layers, the energy source, and the melting material. Identified additive manufacturing methods are: material extrusion, material jetting, vat photopolymerization, powder bed fusion, sheet lamination, binder jetting, and directed energy deposition. Among these, material extrusion and binder jetting are utilized in tissue engineering. Table 1 details the features of the most commonly used 3D printing technologies in tissue engineering.

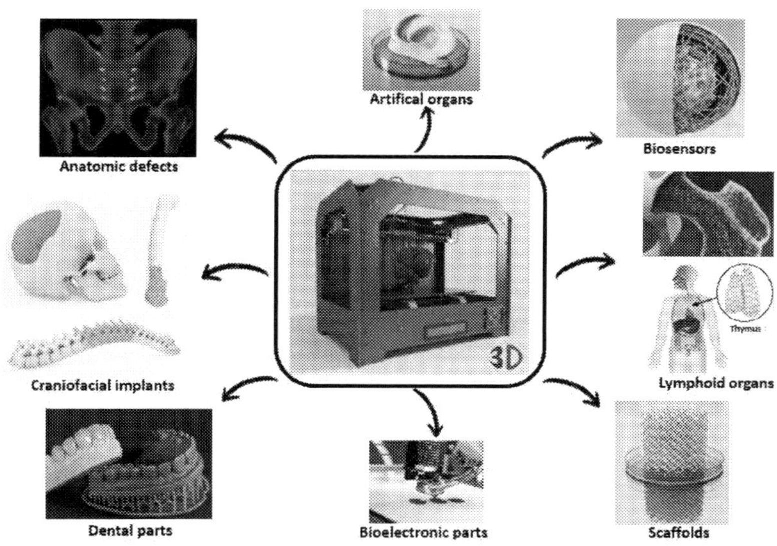

Figure 1. Schematic representation of various biomaterials producedby 3D bioprinting.

Table 1. Types of 3D printing methods for tissue engineering applications (Gittard & Narayan, 2010; Kumar et al., 2019)

3D Printing	Methods	Principle	Parameters	Materials	Advantages	Disadvantages
Material Extrusion	*3D Bioprinting*	The sticky biomaterial contains growth factors and cells. A stepper motor or air pressure is used to extrude a 3D structure.	The thickness of a layer = 40-1000 μm.	A mixture of polymeric biomaterials and cells or extracellular matrix material can generate the tissue analog.	Various biomaterials can be used as long as they can be extruded at physiological temperature. Low initial and running costs. Simply recognizable printing method. Easily operated process of material change.	Visible layer lines. There may be a need for assistance. Weak part durability along Z-axis (perpendicular to build platform). Printing time is increased by more acceptable resolution and a larger print area.
	Fused deposition modeling	To create the 3D structure, a thermoplastic fiber is extruded through a heated nozzle.	The thickness of a layer = 250-370 μm.	Polymer.	Low cost, Less complex, Easy ergonomics, Compact design.	Rough surface finishing, Longer printing time, Limited to thermoplastic polymers.
Binder Jetting	*3D Powder Printing*	A powder-based material and a binder are used in the jetting process. Between the powder layers, the binder acts as an adhesive. The binder is usually liquid, while the build material is typically a powder. To build the layer, this ink binds the powder particles.	The thickness of a layer = 20-100 μm (Parameters depend on the powder particle size and shape).	Metals, ceramics, polymers, and composites are just a few materials used as powder.	It has a very high production speed, extensive size capabilities, and a low-cost method for 3D printing the ability to process a wide range of materials.	High cost of systems, Additional post-processing (Such as heat treatment) can add significant time to the overall process.

Mostly, printable biomaterials such as polymers (synthetic and natural), bioinks, or hydrogels, must have sufficient viscosity to be printable as well as structurally robust, can design 3D structures in a matter of minutes, have the potential to be mechanically reinforced through the application of UV irradiation, chemical cross-linking, or biological, have controllable mechanical properties, have sufficient degradation kinetics, be biomimetic, be biocompatible, and be able to inspect release molecules or drugs (Mobaraki et al., 2020). Also, biomaterial inks should be easily manufactured, shaped, and economically available. For these reasons, a balance must be struck between these characteristics to achieve 3D printed biomaterials with robust qualities for biomedical applications. In this sense, the 3D printing method is an advisable technology for producing customized medicines, thus developing patient conformity by adapting the treatment. Furthermore, on-demand manufacturing in the clinical context can be used (Raijada et al., 2021).

Therefore, this book chapter will present a complete overview of the currently available 3D-printable materials, examining their key benefits, current limits, and possible applications in medicine and tissue engineering. I hope that this chapter will be of assistance and inspiration to the scientific community in moving forward with the possible creation of 3D printing materials.

Polymer Inks

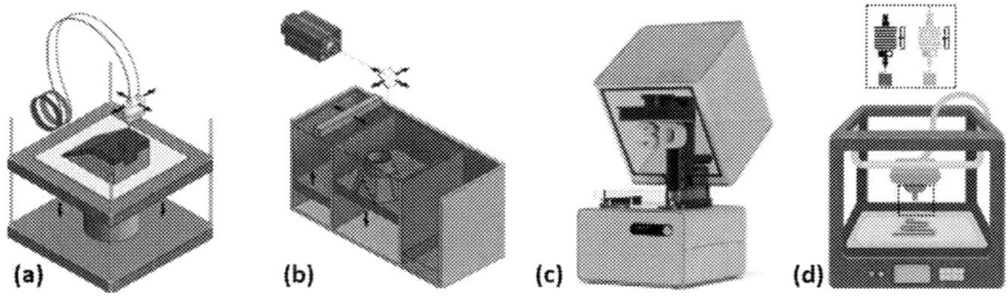

Figure 2. A Schematic diagram for the representation of 3D printing techniques (a) Fused deposition modeling (FDM), (b) Powder-beads for selective laser sintering (SLS), (c) Solutions for stereolithography (SLA), and (d) Direct ink writing (DIW).

The most common biomaterials 3D printing technologies that mainly use polymer filaments are fused deposition modeling (FDM). In addition, solutions for stereolithography (SLA), additive manufacturing of powder beads for selective laser sintering (SLS), and gels/pasty materials for direct ink writing (DIW). A schematic diagram for the representation of 3D printing techniques is shown in Figure 2. The notable advantages of biopolymers, such as controllable degradation, attractive biocompatibility, and mechanical properties, provide a wide range of opportunities for their utilization as printable inks (Ligon et al., 2017).

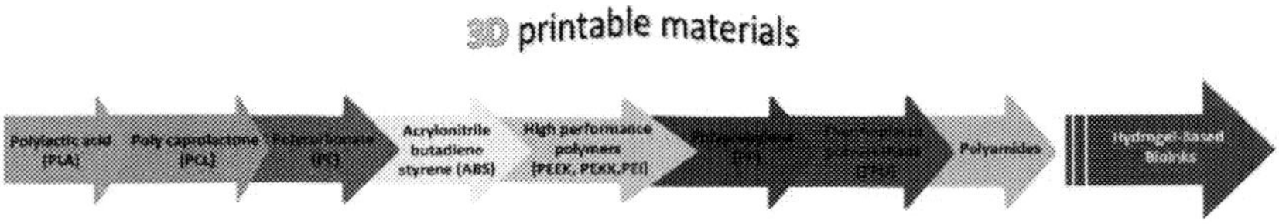

Figure 3. Polymeric materials are most widely used in 3D printing techniques.

The polymeric materials (Figure 3) and properties most widely used in 3D printing techniques are explained below. Also, the chemical structures of the described polymer materials are given in Table 2.

Table 2. Functional 3D printed polymeric materials (Wypych, 2016)

Polylactic acid (PLA) 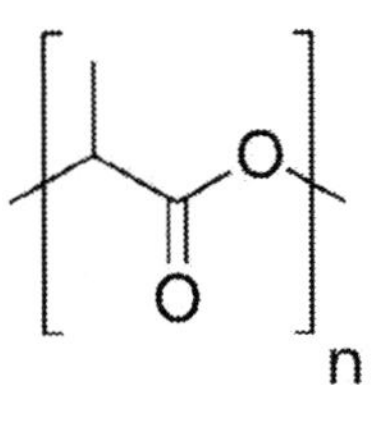	*Polycaprolactone (PCL)* 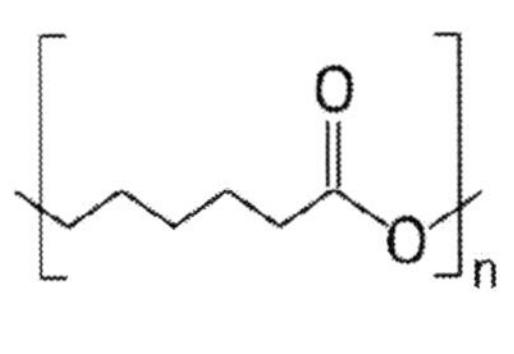	*Acrylonitrile butadiene styrene (ABS)* 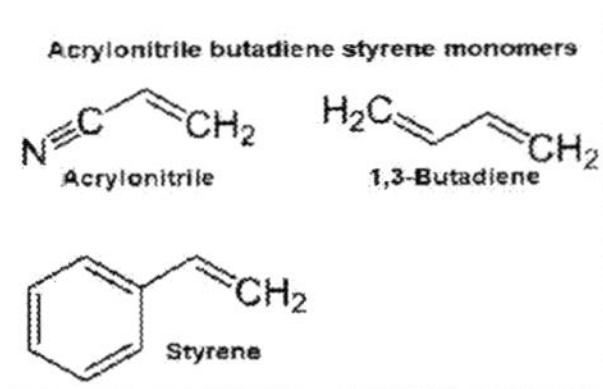
Polycarbonate (PC) 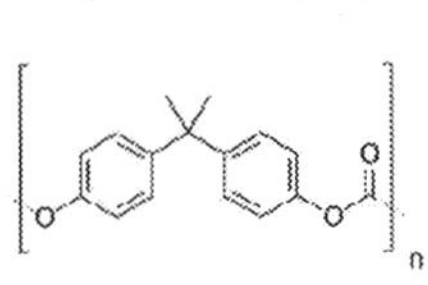	*Polyetheretherketone (PEEK)* 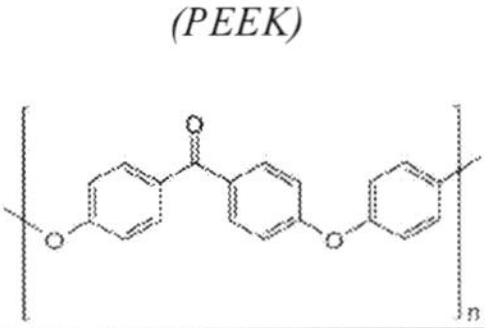	*Polyetherketoneketone (PEKK)* 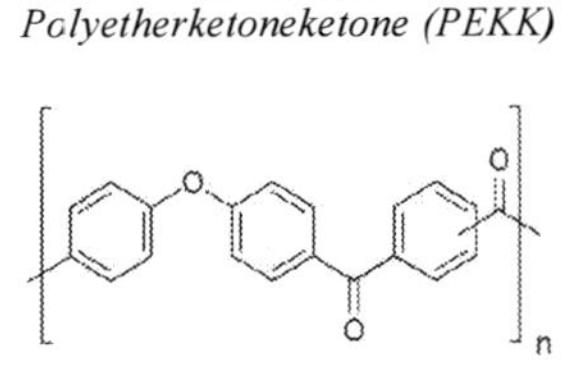

Polyetherimide (PEI) 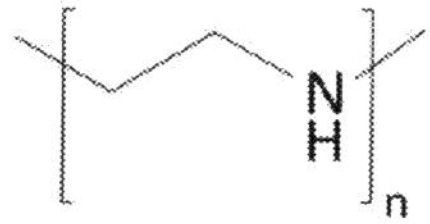	*Thermoplastic polyurethane (TPU)* 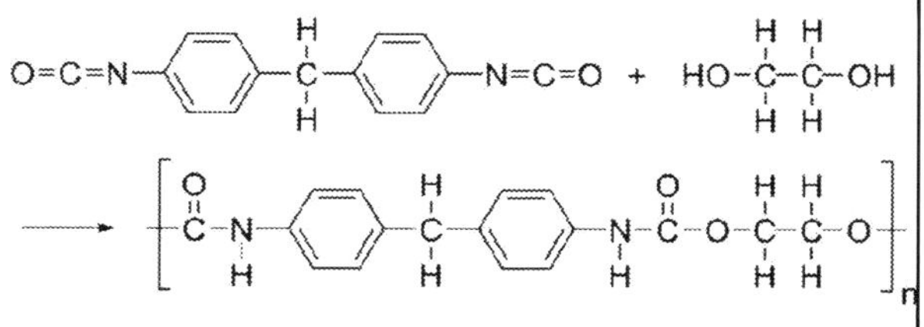 The urethane groups –NH–(C=O)–O– join the molecular units in the Polyurethane synthesis.
Polypropylene (PP) 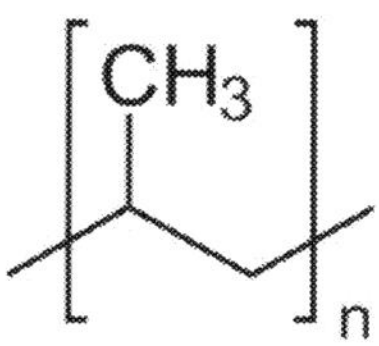	*Polyamides (Kevlar structure chain)* 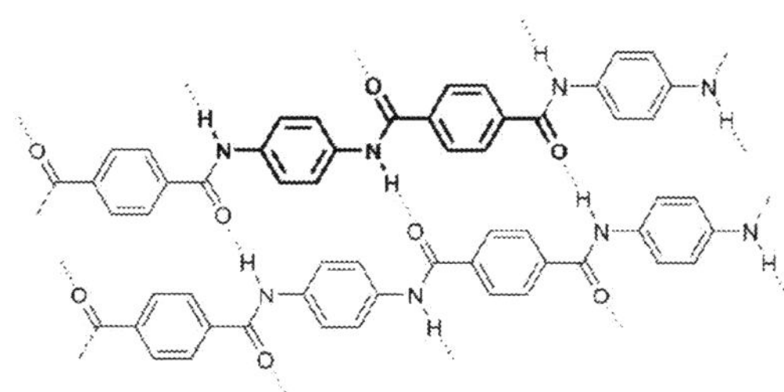

Polylactic Acid (PLA)

Because of the ester linkages that connect the monomer units, polylactic acid (PLA) is categorized as an aliphatic polyester. Also, poly (lactic acid) is biocompatible and biodegradable, and a hydrolysis reaction can readily break it down. It has a wide range of biomedical applications, including resorbable sutures, scaffolds for tissue engineering surgical/ophthalmic implants, and controlled drug-delivery systems. Thermoplastic monomer PLA is extracted from renewable, organic sources such as sugar cane or corn starch and can be efficiently extruded between 190°C and 230°C (PLA, T_m is around *175°C*). PLA is an accessible material to work with and combine in various compounds and remains the most popular polymeric material for 3D printing of FDM (Da Silva et al., 2018).

An important aspect of PLA for medical applications is long-term biocompatibility (at 37°C, ≈ 3-5 years in a saline environment and when UTS PLA 50%, between 6 to 12 months in a saline environment at 37°C) and biodegradability (Sin et al., 2012). PLA is destroyed by a process known as hydrolysis. During this reaction, acidic by-products are released that can affect long-term biocompatibility. These acid derivatives could lead to tissue inflammation and cell death (Arora et al., 2018; Shebi & Lisa, 2018).

Furthermore, hydrophobic PLA surfaces promote bacterial adhesion and the formation of biofilms (Martin et al., 2019). To solve this problem, PLA can be combined with calcium phosphate-based ceramics to increase bone responsiveness and decrease localized acidic environment production (Schiller & Epple, 2003). In addition, the degradation rate of PLA is modified when copolymerized with PLLA. PLA combines with PLLA, prolonging the degeneration time because D-lactic acid is complex for enzymes to degrade in the *in vivo* environment (Woodruff & Hutmacher, 2010).

Despite these disadvantages, PLA has favorable mechanical properties (especially compressive strength) comparable to bone (cortical *bone* ≈100-230 MPa), making it ideal for musculoskeletal tissue engineering. Furthermore, developing PLA-based composites with ceramics/additives can also be advantageous in modifying and increasing the compressive strength and elasticity of the implanted material. These acquired properties allow PLA biocomposites to be used as orthopedic support materials (Bagaria et al., 2018).

Polycaprolactone (PCL)

PCL is a low-cost and biodegradable polyester similar to PLA, having a low melting temperature of 60°C and a glass transition temperature of around −60°C. PCL is synthesized by ring-opening polymerization of ε-caprolactone using a catalyst such as stannous octanoate. PCL is degraded under physiological conditions (e.g., in the human body) by hydrolysis of its ester bonds and has therefore received considerable attention for use as an implantable biomaterial. Compared to other aliphatic polyesters, PCL is easy to fabricate and process into various three-dimensional platforms due to its excellent rheological and viscoelastic properties. (Especially with the emergence of fused deposition modeling (FDM)). PCL has excellent viscoelastic and rheological properties when heated, (e.g., $E = 216$ MPa, $\varepsilon = 746\%$, $\sigma = 37$ MPa), making it a prime candidate for FDM printing to produce longer-term degradable implants (Eshraghi & Das, 2010).

PCL is stable in an *in vivo* environment for more than six months and degrades fully in around three years, depending on molecular weight, crystallinity degree, and degradation conditions. Therefore, as with PLA, it can aid in healing or tissue regeneration and is subsequently biodegraded without releasing potentially toxic by-products (Dziadek et al., 2015; Woodruff & Hutmacher, 2010). Furthermore, the degradation time of PCL is longer than that of poly (lactic acid) or poly (glycolic acid), making it more applicable for long-term medical devices, such as drug delivery systems with a half-life of more than a year. In addition, PCL is a good candidate for scaffold fabrication with powder-beads for selective laser sintering and direct ink writing because it forms strongly cross-linked nanofibers and microfibers, resulting in a macroscale scaffold with enough porosity for growth factors, drugs, embedding cells, and so on (Williams et al., 2005).

Polycarbonate (PC)

Polycarbonate is a high-performance, amorphous, durable, and transparent thermoplastic polymer with organic functional groups connected by carbonate groups (–O–(C=O)–O–). These properties exhibit an inimitable combination. Moreover, PC is renowned as an engineering plastic because of its unique features, such as excellent dimensional stability, high impact strength, and good electrical properties.

Polycarbonate is a transparent superior plastic and its glass transition temperature is nearly 150°C, so above this point, it gradually softens and flows above about 155°C. Although the main properties of polycarbonate are similar to those of acrylic and polymethyl methacrylate (PMMA), polycarbonate is more substantial and can be used in a broader range of temperatures (Rokicki & Parzuchowski, 2012).

In recent years, PC has been used as a blood oxygenator, blood reservoir and orthopedic scaffolds for medical applications, as it has tunable mechanical properties with Young's modulus, tensile strength, flexural strength, and elongation of 2370 MPa, 65 MPa, 93 MPa, and 110%, respectively (De la Colina-Martínez et al., 2017). Due to the unique set of chemical and physical properties of PC are used extensively in fused deposition modeling 3D printing to produce stable, strong plastic products with a high melting point. Apart from all these promising properties, polycarbonate is relatively tricky for amateurs to print on compared to thermoplastics such as acrylonitrile butadiene styrene (ABS) or polylactic acid (PLA) because it has a high melting point, adheres poorly to the print bed, warps during printing, and at the same time PC tends to absorb moisture from the air. *These negative* tendencies can influence 3D printing performance and strength. Despite these problems, 3D polycarbonate printing is widely used by professional users (Hacker et al., 2019).

Acrylonitrile Butadiene Styrene (ABS)

Acrylonitrile Butadiene Styrene is an impact-resistant engineering thermoplastic and amorphous polymer with the chemical formula $((C_8H_8)_x\cdot(C_4H_6)_y\cdot(C_3H_3N)_z)$. ABS is synthesized with the polymerization of styrene and acrylonitrile in the existence of polybutadiene. ABS copolymer is an ideal thermoplastic material with good durability and elasticity, high stiffness, and good impact resistance. In addition, it has good abrasion and elongation resistance and high dimensional stability (mechanically solid and stable over time). It also has good insulating properties even at low temperatures. Furthermore, ABS exhibits the appropriate combination of thermal, electrical, and mechanical properties, a high degree of surface brightness/quality, and excellent surface aspects (Khanna, 2021).

Pure ABS polymers are vulnerable to oxidizing chemicals and strong acids, and in the presence of certain organic compounds, they may experience stress corrosion cracking. ABS shows poor resistance to alcohols, halogenated hydrocarbons, aromatic hydrocarbons, and UV light degrades ABS unless certain additives are incorporated. In addition, ABS has disadvantages like poor weathering resistance, low dielectric strength, and low continuous service temperature. Despite these disadvantages, ABS can withstand temperatures from −20°C to 80°C without any problems. ABS with a melting temperature of 105°C, ABS becomes an attractive alternative for fused deposition modeling and solutions for stereolithography systems. Acrylonitrile Butadiene Styrene is widely used as an *orthotics and cartilage tissue* biomaterial for 3D printing, as it is a strong and not biodegradable thermoplastic (Rosenzweig et al., 2015).

High-Performance Polymers

Polyetheretherketone (PEEK)

Polyaryletheretherketone (PAEK), often known as PEEK, is a PAEK polymer family commonly utilized in orthopedic spinal implants. PEEK is a polycyclic, semi-crystalline, linear, aromatic thermoplastic having an aromatic molecular backbone connected between aryl rings by ketone and ether functional groups.

Because of this chemical structure, PEEKs exhibit desirable physical properties and durability against environmental challenges. At standard ambient temperature, Polyetheretherketone is chemically inert and insoluble in all common solvents except 98% H_2SO_4. PEEK can be dissolved entirely only with rather esoteric solvents, such as diaryl sulfones. As for its mechanical behavior, the compressive modulus, the flexural modulus, and the tensile modulus of PEEK are ≈ 2.8, 3.6, 3.8 GPa, respectively. PEEK maintains stability at high temperatures and is resistant to chemical and radiation damage. The glass transition temperature of PEEK is 145°C and a crystalline melt transition temperature of around 343°C.

Furthermore, in clinical practice, gamma irradiation at dosages of 25–40 kGy can be utilized to sterilize PEEK in the air (Kurtz, 2012; Kurtz & Devine, 2007). Since then, PEEK has been widely used in trauma, orthopedics, spine, and dental implants. Polyetherketoneketone (PEKK), another principal constituent of PAEK, has lately been widely explored as a possible orthopedic implant. PEEK scaffolds with controllable pore sizes have been created using 3D printing processes such as fused filament fabrication and selective laser sintering due to superior chemical resistance, radiolucency, and mechanical properties similar to human bones (Spece et al., 2020).

Polyetherketoneketone (PEKK)

Polyetherketoneketone (PEKK) and polyetheretherketone (PEEK) are the two best known members of the polyaryletherketone (PAEK) family. The polyether ketone ketone (PEKK) is a methacrylate-free, semi-crystalline, high-performance thermoplastic material. It is a novel polymer material that has attracted the consideration of scientists due to its excellent biological, mechanical, and physical properties that can be used in many biomedical applications. PEEK and PEKK have aromatic rings that differ in the ratio of the ether and ketone groups.

There are various distinctions between PEKK and PEEK. The second ketone group in PEKK polymers stiffens the backbone chain and polarity, increasing the melting temperature and glass transition. Furthermore, PEKK has amorphous and crystalline properties, creating a wide range of products. For example, a PEKK with 60% straight and 40% kinked segments melts at 305°C, whereas a PEEK with 80% straight and 20% kinked segments melts at 360°C. Furthermore, the additional ketone group in PEKK has more robust polymer chains and superior physical and mechanical properties, such as melting temperature and compressive strength, than other polymeric materials.

Moreover, compared to other polymeric materials, the extra ketone group in PEKK has more robust polymer chains and higher physical and mechanical properties, such as compressive strength and melting temperature. Compared to PEEK, PEKK exhibits superior mechanical properties in terms of flexure strength (140–200 MPa), tensile strength (115 MPa), compressive strength (246 MPa), and elastic modulus (5.1 GPa). Dental implants, temporary abutments, fixed prostheses, removable dentures, finger prostheses, and restorative material in fixed prosthetics are among the promising applications of the PEEK biomaterial. Fused deposition modeling, the most common 3D printing technology, has been used to fabricate personalized PEKK parts (Alqurashi et al., 2021; Cheng et al., 2020).

Ultem® (Polyetherimide, PEI)

Ultem is a family of polyetherimide thermoplastics with excellent mechanical and thermal properties. Polyetherimide (PEI) is an amber-colored, amorphous, translucent thermoplastic with similar properties to PEEK. The repeating unit of polyetherimide has the chemical formula $C_{37}H_{24}O_6N_2$. PEI has a glass transition temperature of 217°C. In chlorinated solvents, it is prone to stress cracking. PEI is less expensive than PEEK. However, it has a lower impact strength. Polyetherimide can withstand high temperatures with stable electrical properties over a wide frequency range (Ultem 1000, thermal conductivity 0.122 W/m·K - 0.22 W/m·K). Ultem has good strength and stiffness and can survive continuous use at temperatures up to 171°C. It is easily machined and manufactured. This high-strength material has exceptional chemical resistance and ductility, making it more suitable for many applications. Due to its adhesive properties and chemical stability, it can be additively manufactured using fused deposition modeling, a method in which parts are deposited layer by layer by extrusion. Ultem resins are used in medical and healthcare devices such as sterilization trays, stopcocks, dental types of equipment, and pipettes because of their solvent resistance, flame resistance, and heat resistance. In recent years, polyetherimide seems an exciting material for producing membranes in biohybrid organ systems and endoprosthetic replacement applications (Lau, 2014).

Polypropylene (PP)

Polypropylene (PP), commonly known as polypropene, is considered one of the lightest and most versatile crystalline thermoplastic polymers. It is made through chain-growth polymerization from the monomer propylene, which has a melting point of 165°C. Polypropylene is a partly crystalline and non-polar polyolefin polymer. It has comparable properties to polyethylene; however, it is more heat resistant and more robust. Polypropylene can be manufactured using a variety of processes, including injection molding and extrusion. It is a free-color material with excellent mechanical properties (The elastic modulus of PP is between 1300-1800 N/mm^2) and is better than polyethylene. Polypropylene has strength at break (20-40 MPa) and a crystalline structure with high stiffness (1.2-1.6 GPa) compared to other commercial thermoplastics. Polypropylene has poor resistance to halogenated hydrocarbons and aromatic compounds.

On the other hand, it has good resistance to aldehydes, aliphatic hydrocarbons, alcohols, esters, and strong chemical resistance to dilute and concentrated acids and ketones (Hisham A. Maddah, 2016). Its primary disadvantage is its low-temperature resistance (brittleness below −20°C) and susceptibility to UV light, which causes it to enlarge and swell quickly in aromatic and chlorinated solvents. Nonetheless, polypropylene is widely used to make personalized 3D-printed orthotics for fractures, reusable plastic containers, non-absorbable sutures, and pharmacy prescription bottles because of its lightweight and rigidity (Wang et al., 2018).

Thermoplastic Polyurethane (TPU)

TPU is a polyurethane material with qualities ranging from high-performance elastomer to tough thermoplastic. It is frequently utilized due to its excellent physical attributes and chemical structural adaptability. Thermoplastic polyurethane is a linear block copolymer with alternating hard and soft segments. The hard segment comprises alternating diisocyanates with short-chain diols, while diisocyanates form the soft segment with long-chain diols. TPU has various advantages such as transparency, elasticity, grease and abrasion, resistance to oil, ability to operate at low temperatures, mechanical properties, and rubber-like elasticity. The TPU has variable mechanical characteristics, having an elastic modulus range between 5 to 100 MPa and a break elongation of 300%. TPU powders are also utilized in other 3D printing methods, including selective laser sintering and 3D inkjet printing. It is also used in oversized vertical injection molding or extrusion molding machines to print directly without an intermediary step such as filament extrusion or powder preparation. TPU offers a wide range of applications, including automobile instrument panels, drive belts, flexible yet durable orthotic and medical devices, and a wide range of extruded films, sheets, and profiles for biomedical applications (Feng & Ye, 2011; Van Alsenoy et al., 2019).

Polyamides

Polyamides (PA, often known as nylon) are significant thermoplastic polymers with an amide linkage (–NH–C=O) in their backbone. Polyamides generally include proteins and peptides, naturally produced polymers composed of repeating amino acid units. Proteins are examples of naturally occurring polyamides. Polyamides are classified into several categories, depending on their monomer arrangement and chemical composition. Aromatic (Kevlar© and plastics produced from carbamide), cycloaliphatic (Cycloaliphatic epoxy resins such as bisphenol) and aliphatic polyamides (they are also known as *nylons)* are essential types of polyamides. Polyamides are usually used with powder beads for selective laser sintering. However, some modifications, such as nylon, are also available for fused deposition modeling. Polyamides offer an excellent combination of chemical and mechanical properties (Ultimate *tensile strength is* 10 MPa) with good thermal resistance (some nylon have a melting point of ≈ 300°C), high abrasion, and good fatigue resistance. In addition, polyamides containing polar groups in the molecular chain have high biocompatibility with human tissue, owing to their chemical structure and active groups' resemblance to collagen protein. Therefore, they can be combined with nano-hydroxyapatite particles (n-HA) as porous scaffolds for orthopedic applications (Khadka et al., 2011).

Dynamic Hydrogels in 3D Printing

Hydrogels are three-dimensional networks of cross-linked hydrophilic polymer chains with a high water content and a wide range of biophysical properties. Reversible non-covalent interactions, also known as supramolecular contacts, are caused by the dynamic behavior of polymer chains and include metal-ligand coordination, hydrogen bonding, π-π interaction, electrostatic interaction, hydrophobic interaction, and Van der Waals forces (Heidarian et al., 2019). Because of their biocompatibility, tunable mechanics, and disintegration, hydrogels are suitable soft material systems for imitating the natural microenvironment of the extracellular matrix

(ECM). Hydrogels can also be functionalized after injection into the living organism with specific molecules that attract and bind growth factors. For instance, heparin-functionalized amphiphile peptide hydrogels attract angiogenic growth factors including TGF-1, VEGF, BDNF, IGF-1 and fibroblast growth factor 2 (FGF2), which promote blood vessel regeneration (Prince & Kumacheva, 2019; Rajangam et al., 2006). Figure 4 shows a schematic representation of the technique to produce injectable hydrogels for cartilage and bone tissue engineering applications.

Hydrogels are intriguing because they can be designed to mimic the extracellular tissue microenvironment, allowing them to be used in medicine as scaffolds for tissue regeneration, biosensors, and drug delivery systems. To satisfy the needs of the end product, hydrogels can be formed and printed in a range of forms, sizes, and embodiments (Kamata et al., 2015). Chemical and photo-crosslinking provide the most stable and mechanically adjustable hydrogels. Polymerization of the bioink occurs after extrusion in photo-crosslinking and does not affect the viscosity of the bioink (Lim et al., 2020). There have been several attempts to use 3D printing to create complex biological structures from hydrogels. For instance, fibrin, alginate, and gelatin were previously used to create 3D printed hydrogels. Hydrogel and polymer-based inks can be printed using a variety of processes, including inkjet, extrusion, laser-assisted bioprinting, and stereolithography (Li et al., 2018).

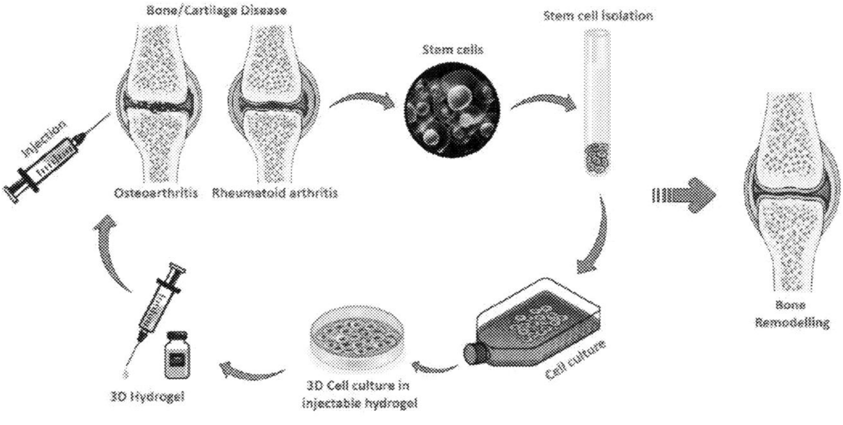

Figure 4. Schematic representation of the technique for producing injectable hydrogels for cartilage and tissue engineering applications.

Conclusion

Unlike traditional manufacturing technologies, which are time-consuming or material-intensive, 3D printing allows for the controlled layer-by-layer deposition of predetermined items. 3D printing is a computer-aided manufacturing process to produce 3D objects/materials with complex geometries in regenerative medicine, tissue engineering, orthotic devices, defect modeling, and drug systems. Despite several significant breakthroughs in this subject/field, there are still certain hurdles for future technology development. The fundamental problem is creating high-performance biomaterials with good chemical and mechanical characteristics to create regenerative implants while also fully replicating the biological functioning and structural complexity of the original tissues/organs. Tissue engineering, materials engineering, and medical researchers may use 3D bioprinting technology to 3D print physiologically relevant structures using biomaterial-based bioinks. Several of these biomaterials have exhibited greater strength and durability compared to the original tissue or organ.

Polymer-based inks have received a lot of attention since they can be used in various printing methods and have excellent mechanical properties. The biocompatibility of raw materials with cellular growth, cell proliferation, and printing properties like viscosity, extrudability, and mechanical stability substantially impact the selection of raw materials for 3D bioprinting. However, substantial limits remain for the future development of such biomaterials, including their long-term biocompatibility, protracted degradation time, and absence of bioactive signals for cell attachment and proliferation. Thus, basic knowledge and integration of the biological microenvironment with materials science are necessary to create a novel bioink and fabricate 3D bioprinting tissue structures.

In this context, tremendous progress in the fabrication of printed hydrogels has been made in recent years. As mentioned in this book chapter, these materials are appropriate because they produce biomimetic microenvironments capable of directing cells. Therefore, further research in bioprinting and biomaterials technology will bring 3D printing closer to creating life-size, fully functional 3D-printed tissues/organs.

References

Ahlfeld, T., Lode, A., Richter, R. F., Pradel, W., Franke, A., Rauner, M., Stadlinger, B.,

Lauer, G., Gelinsky, M., Korn, P., & Henningsen, A. (2021). Toward biofabrication of resorbable implants consisting of a calcium phosphate cement and fibrin-a characterization *in vitro* and *in vivo*. *International Journal of Molecular Sciences Article Int. J. Mol. Sci*, *22*, 1–16. https://doi.org/10.3390/ijms22031218.

Alqurashi, H., Khurshid, Z., Syed, A. U. Y., Rashid Habib, S., Rokaya, D., & Zafar, M. S. (2021). Polyetherketoneketone (PEKK): An emerging biomaterial for oral implants and dental prostheses. *Journal of Advanced Research*, 28, 87–95. https://doi.org/10.1016/j.jare.2020.09.004.

Arora, B., Bhatia, R., & Attri, P. (2018). Bionanocomposites: Green materials for a sustainable future. In C. M. Hussain & A. K. Mishra (Eds.), *New Polymer Nanocomposites for Environmental Remediation* (pp. 699–712). Elsevier Inc. https://doi.org/10.1016/B978-0-12-811033-1.00027-5.

Bagaria, V., Bhansali, R., & Pawar, P. (2018). 3D printing- creating a blueprint for the future of orthopedics: Current concept review and the road ahead! *Journal of Clinical Orthopaedics and Trauma*, 9 (3), 207–212. https://doi.org/10.1016/j.jcot.2018.07.007.

Cheng, K. jie, Liu, Y. feng, Wang, R., Zhang, J. xing, Jiang, X. feng, Dong, X. tao, & Xu, X. (2020). Topological optimization of 3D printed bone analog with PEKK for surgical mandibular reconstruction. *Journal of the Mechanical Behavior of Biomedical Materials*, 107, 1–9. https://doi.org/10.1016/j.jmbbm.2020.103758.

Chu, T., Wang, H., Qiu, Y., Luo, H., He, B., Wu, B., & Gao, B. (2021). 3D printed smart silk wearable sensors. *Analyst*, 146 (5), 1552–1558. https://doi.org/10.1039/d0an02292f.

Da Silva, D., Kaduri, M., Poley, M., Adir, O., Krinsky, N., Shainsky-Roitman, J., & Schroeder, A. (2018). Biocompatibility, biodegradation, and excretion of polylactic acid (PLA) in medical implants and theranostic systems. *Chemical Engineering Journal*, 340, 9–14. https://doi.org/10.1016/j.cej.2018.01.010.

De la Colina-Martínez, A. L., Martínez-Barrera, G., Barrera-Díaz, C. E., ávila-Córdoba, L. I., & Ureña-Núñez, F. (2017). Characterization of recycled polycarbonate from electronic waste and its use in hydraulic concrete: Improvement of compressive performance. *Advances in Concrete Construction*, *5* (6), 563–573. https://doi.org/10.12989/acc.2017.5.6.563.

Dziadek, M., Pawlik, J., Menaszek, E., Stodolak-Zych, E., & Cholewa-Kowalska, K. (2015). Effect of the preparation methods on architecture, crystallinity, hydrolytic degradation, bioactivity, and biocompatibility of PCL/bioglass composite scaffolds. *Journal of Biomedical Materials Research - Part B Applied Biomaterials*, 103 (8), 1580–1593. https://doi.org/10.1002/jbm.b.33350.

Eshraghi, S., & Das, S. (2010). Mechanical and microstructural properties of polycaprolactone scaffolds with one-dimensional, two-dimensional, and three-dimensional orthogonally oriented porous architectures produced by selective laser sintering. *Acta Biomaterialia*, 6 (7), 2467–2476. https://doi.org/10.1016/j.actbio.2010.02.002.

Feng, F., & Ye, L. (2011). Morphologies and mechanical properties of polylactide/thermoplastic polyurethane elastomer blends. *Journal of Applied Polymer Science*, 119 (5), 2778–2783. https://doi.org/10.1002/app.32863.

Gittard, S. D., & Narayan, R. J. (2010). Laser direct writing of micro-and nano-scale medical devices. *Expert Review of Medical Devices*, 7 (3), 343–356. https://doi.org/10.1586/erd.10.14.

Hacker, M. C., Krieghoff, J., & Mikos, A. G. (2019). Chapter 33 - synthetic polymers. In *Principles of Regenerative Medicine (Third Edition)* (Vol. 2, pp. 587–622). Elsevier Inc.

Heidarian, P., Kouzani, A. Z., Kaynak, A., Paulino, M., & Nasri-Nasrabadi, B. (2019). Dynamic Hydrogels and Polymers as Inks for Three-Dimensional Printing. *ACS Biomaterials Science and Engineering*, *5* (6), 2688–2707. https://doi.org/10.1021/acsbiomaterials.9b00047.

Hisham A. Maddah. (2016). Polypropylene as a promising plastic: a review. *American Journal of Polymer Science*, 6 (1), 1–11. https://doi.org/10.5923/j.ajps.20160601.01

Kamata, H., Li, X., Chung, U., & Sakai, T. (2015). Design of hydrogels for biomedical applications. *Advanced Healthcare Materials*, 4 (16), 2360–2374. https://doi.org/10.1002/adhm.201500076.

Khadka, A., Li, J., Li, Y., Gao, Y., Zuo, Y., & Ma, Y. (2011). Evaluation of hybrid porous biomimetic nano-hydroxyapatite/polyamide 6 and bone marrow-derived stem cell construct in the repair of the calvarial critical-size defect. *Journal of Craniofacial Surgery*, 22 (5), 1852–1858. https://doi.org/10.1097/ SCS.0b013e31822e8274.

Khanna, A. S. (2021). Natural degradation on plastics and corrosion of plastics in industrial environment. In *Reference Module in Materials Science and Materials Engineering* (Vol. 1). Elsevier. https://doi.org/10.1016/b978-0-12-820352-1.00105-x.

Koch, L., Kuhn, S., Sorg, H., Gruene, M., Schlie, S., Gaebel, R., Polchow, B., Reimers, K., Stoelting, S., Ma, N., Vogt, P. M., Steinhoff, G., & Chichkov, B. (2010). Laser printing of skin cells and human stem cells. *Tissue Engineering - Part C: Methods*, 16 (5), 847–854. https://doi.org/10.1089/ten.tec.2009.0397.

Kolesky, D. B., Truby, R. L., Gladman, A. S., Busbee, T. A., Homan, K. A., & Lewis, J. A. (2014). Bioprinting: 3D bioprinting of vascularized, heterogeneous cell-laden tissue constructs. *Advanced Materials*, 26 (19), 3124–3130. https://doi.org/10.1002/adma.201470124.

Kumar, A., Ahlawat, J., & Narayan, M. (2019). 3D bioprinting for organs, skin, and engineered tissues. In *3D Printing Technology in Nanomedicine* (pp. 115–128). Elsevier. https://doi.org/10.1016/B978-0-12-815890-6.00006-2.

Kurtz, S. M. (2012). Chemical and Radiation Stability of PEEK. In *PEEK Biomaterials Handbook* (pp. 75–79). Elsevier. https://doi.org/10.1016/B978-1-4377-4463-7.10006-5.

Kurtz, S. M., & Devine, J. N. (2007). PEEK biomaterials in trauma, orthopedic, and spinal implants. In *Biomaterials*, 28 (32), 4845–4869. https://doi.org/10.1016/j.biomaterials.2007.07.013.

Lau, K. S. Y. (2014). High-performance polyimides and high-temperature resistant polymers. In *Handbook of Thermoset Plastics* (Vol. 3, pp. 297–424). Elsevier. https://doi.org/10.1016/B978-1-4557-3107-7.00010-5.

Li, H., Tan, C., & Li, L. (2018). Review of 3D printable hydrogels and constructs. *Materials and Design*, 159, 20–38. https://doi.org/10.1016/j.matdes.2018.08.023.

Ligon, S. C., Liska, R., Stampfl, J., Gurr, M., & Mülhaupt, R. (2017). Polymers for 3D printing and customized additive manufacturing. *Chemical Reviews*, 117 (15), 10212–10290. https://doi.org/10.1021/acs.chemrev.7b00074.

Lim, K. S., Galarraga, J. H., Cui, X., Lindberg, G. C. J., Burdick, J. A., & Woodfield, T. B. F. (2020). Fundamentals and applications of photo-cross-linking in bioprinting. *Chemical Reviews*, 120 (19), 10662–10694. https://doi.org/10.1021/ acs.chemrev.9 b00812.

Martin, V., Ribeiro, I. A., Alves, M. M., Gonçalves, L., Claudio, R. A., Grenho, L., Fernandes, M. H., Gomes, P., Santos, C. F., & Bettencourt, A. F. (2019). Engineering a multifunctional 3D-printed PLA-collagen-minocycline-nano-Hydroxyapatite scaffold with combined antimicrobial and osteogenic effects for bone regeneration. *Materials Science and Engineering C*, 101, 15–26. https://doi.org/10.1016/j.msec.2019.03.056.

Mobaraki, M., Ghaffari, M., Yazdanpanah, A., Luo, Y., & Mills, D. K. (2020). Bioinks and bioprinting: A focused review. *Bioprinting*, 18, 1–16. https://doi.org/10.1016/j.bprint.2020.e00080.

Prince, E., & Kumacheva, E. (2019). Design and applications of man-made biomimetic fibrillar hydrogels. *Nature Reviews Materials*, 4 (2), 99–115. https://doi.org/10.1038/s41578-018-0077-9.

Raijada, D., Wac, K., Greisen, E., Rantanen, J., & Genina, N. (2021). Integration of personalized drug delivery systems into digital health. *Advanced Drug Delivery Reviews*, 176, 1–19. https://doi.org/10.1016/j.addr.2021.113857.

Rajangam, K., Behanna, H. A., Hui, M. J., Han, X., Hulvat, J. F., Lomasney, J. W., & Stupp, S. I. (2006). Heparin-binding nanostructures to promote the growth of blood vessels. *Nano Letters*, 6 (9), 2086–2090. https://doi.org/10.1021/nl0613555.

Rokicki, G., & Parzuchowski, P. G. (2012). ROP of cyclic carbonates and ROP of macrocycles. In *Polymer Science: A Comprehensive Reference* (4th ed., Vol. 4, pp. 247–308). Elsevier Inc. https://doi.org/10.1016/B978-0-444-53349-4.00107-2.

Rosenzweig, D. H., Carelli, E., Steffen, T., Jarzem, P., & Haglund, L. (2015). 3D-printed ABS and PLA scaffolds for cartilage and nucleus pulpous tissue regeneration. *International Journal of Molecular Sciences*, 16 (7), 15118–15135. https://doi.org/10.3390/ijms160715118.

Sachlos, E., Czernuszka, J. T., Gogolewski, S., & Dalby, M. (2003). Making tissue engineering scaffolds work. Review on the application of solid freeform fabrication technology to the production of tissue engineering scaffolds. *European Cells and Materials*, 5, 29–40. https://doi.org/10.22203/ecm.v005a03.

Said, S., Boulkaibet, I., Sheikh, M., Karar, A. S., Alkork, S., & Nait-Ali, A. (2020). Machine-learning-based muscle control of a 3D-printed bionic arm. *Sensors (Switzerland)*, 20 (11), 1–16. https://doi.org/10.3390/s20113144.

Schiller, C., & Epple, M. (2003). Carbonated calcium phosphates are suitable pH-stabilising fillers for biodegradable polyesters. *Biomaterials*, 24 (12), 2037–2043. https://doi.org/10.1016/S0142-9612(02)00634-8.

Shebi, A., & Lisa, S. (2018). Pectin mediated synthesis of nano hydroxyapatite-decorated poly(lactic acid) honeycomb membranes for tissue engineering. *Carbohydrate Polymers*, 201, 39–47. https://doi.org/10.1016/j.carbpol.2018.08.012.

Sin, L. T., Rahmat, R. R., & Rahman, W. A. W. A. (2012). Polylactic acid: PLA biopolymer technology and applications. In *Polylactic Acid: PLA Biopolymer Technology and Applications*. Elsevier Inc. https://doi.org/10.1016/C2010-0-65966-9.

Spece, H., Yu, T., Law, A. W., Marcolongo, M., & Kurtz, S. M. (2020). 3D printed porous PEEK created via fused filament fabrication for osteoconductive orthopedic surfaces. *Journal of the Mechanical Behavior of Biomedical Materials*, 109, 2–9. https://doi.org/10.1016/j.jmbbm.2020.103850.

Van Alsenoy, K., Ryu, J. H., & Girard, O. (2019). The effect of EVA and TPU custom foot orthoses on running economy, running mechanics, and comfort. *Frontiers in Sports and Active Living*, 1. https://doi.org/10.3389/fspor.2019.00034.

Wang, L., Sanders, J. E., Gardner, D. J., & Han, Y. (2018). Effect of fused deposition modeling process parameters on the mechanical properties of a filled polypropylene. *Progress in Additive Manufacturing*, 3 (4), 205–214. https://doi.org/10.1007/s40964-018-0053-3.

Williams, J. M., Adewunmi, A., Schek, R. M., Flanagan, C. L., Krebsbach, P. H., Feinberg, S. E., Hollister, S. J., & Das, S. (2005). Bone tissue engineering using polycaprolactone scaffolds fabricated via selective laser sintering. *Biomaterials*, 26 (23), 4817–4827. https://doi.org/10.1016/j.biomaterials.2004.11.057.

Woodruff, M. A., & Hutmacher, D. W. (2010). The return of a forgotten polymer-Polycaprolactone in the 21st century. *Progress in Polymer Science (Oxford)*, 35 (10), 1217–1256. https://doi.org/10.1016/j.progpolymsci.2010.04.002.

Wypych, G. (2016). Handbook of polymers. In *Handbook of Polymers* (Vol. 2). ChemTec Publishing. https://doi.org/10.1016/c2015-0-01462-9.

Yang, Y., Li, H., Xu, Y., Dong, Y., Shan, W., & Shen, J. (2019). Fabrication and evaluation of dental fillers using customized molds via 3D printing technology. *International Journal of Pharmaceutics*, 562, 66–75. https://doi.org/10.1016/j.ijpharm.2019.03.024.

Chapter 3

New Generation Cell Culture

Emine Tural*, MD
Department of Histology and Embryology,
School of Medicine, Medeniyet University,
Istanbul, Turkey

Abstract

Cells come in many different shapes and sizes. Although most cells are small, some are extremely large. The change in cell size and shape is directly related to the cell's function. Epithelial cells are flat, so they can be tightly packed to protect the body from harmful effects. Longer and thinner muscle cells allow movement by contraction and relaxation. Skin, bone, muscle, and nerve cells are all examples of specialized cells. Although cells come in a wide variety of shapes, sizes, and functions, all cells can be classified into two basic groups, prokaryotic and eukaryotic. Cells have a life cycle of growth, maintenance, and reproduction. The life cycle of most cells is two stages. In the first stage, the cell grows and performs its vital functions. In the second stage, it reproduces itself by cell division.

Despite understanding the pathology and mechanisms of injury of our organs, organ/tissue repair and regeneration studies are still at very early stages. Tissue engineering studies have become increasingly popular in recent years. Tissue products that are naturally derived or engineered from synthetic biocompatible materials are used to replace cells that are problematic or fail to exhibit their normal functional potential. The cell culture method is used in areas such as cell biology, tissue morphology, and engineering, as well as to understand and improve disease mechanisms and drug action.

---

* Corresponding Author's Email: eminetural@gmail.com.

In: Bioprinting the Human
Editors: Soner Şahin and Kenan Demir
ISBN: 978-1-68507-993-2

Cell culture can be two-dimensional and three-dimensional. It is believed that three-dimensional (3D) cell cultures better mimic the *in vivo* environment than two-dimensional (2D) cell cultures. Because the multicellular structure allows cells to interact with each other and with the extracellular matrix (ECM).

Spheroids and organoids are formations closer to natural physiological systems with their three-dimensional structures and have great importance in cancer and stem cell research. Three-dimensional cultures of many organs, such as the brain, kidney, pancreas, stomach, liver, lung, and bladder, have been made so far and have found use in many biomedical applications.

Keywords: spheroids, 3D culture, organoids, cell culture

Introduction

The function of tissues and organs and the mechanisms underlying their disease have become clearer with the use of cell culture systems and animal models (Kapałczyńska et al., 2018). In 1097, Harrison performed the first cell culture to investigate the origin of nerve fibers (Harrison et al., 1907).

Over time, the cell culture process has been developed and used to monitor the growth and differentiation of cells. For cell culture, primary cells isolated directly from the donor or cell lines from cell banks can be used. Cells are isolated from living organisms for use in primary culture and may contain populations of different cell types found in source tissue. Because of this, it is important to isolate the correct cell type. The other alternative cell lines are produced in centers such as ATCC (American Type Culture Collection) for routine use in research (Kapałczyńska et al., 2018).

Cell Culture

Cell culture is one of the fundamental methods for our understanding of the basic biophysical and biomolecular mechanisms by which cells come together in tissues and organs. It has become an indispensable tool to help reveal how tissues work and how their functions are impaired under disease conditions. Cell culture is widely used in medicine, drug studies, tissue engineering, and industrial applications. Since 3D cell culture methods provide more realistic microenvironments, they have started to be used more than 2D cell culture

(Duval et al., 2017a). Cell culture involves the propagation of cells on the appropriate surface in an artificial environment consisting of an ideal source of nutrients, optimum humidity, temperature, and a gas atmosphere. Generally, cells grow in a sterile incubator containing 5% CO at 37°C, within days or weeks (Saji Joseph et al., 2019).

2D Cell Culture

In 2D cell culture, a Petri dish is typically used containing glass or polystyrene structures to attach and provide mechanical support to the cells. It allows the same amount of access to the medium and the growth factors contained in it. As a result, homogeneous growth and proliferation occurs in cells. The advantage of 2D culture is that it is simple to maintain and costs nothing. However, it cannot mimic the natural structures of tissues and tumors (Breslin & O'Driscoll, 2013a; Duval et al., 2017a; Edmondson et al., 2014). Cell-cell and cell extracellular matrix (ECM) relationships cannot be represented as they are *in vivo.* All of these are responsible for cell proliferation, differentiation, viability, expression of proteins, and other cellular functions (Kapałczyńska et al., 2018).

The morphology and division modes of cells change during isolation from tissue and subsequent transfer to 2D culture dishes. Phenotype losses are also a negative effect of 2D cultures. Morphological change can adversely affect the functions of cells, the arrangement of intracellular structures, secretory properties, and cell signaling.

In 2D cell culture, cells have more surface area for contact with plastic and medium, forcing them to polarize that does not reflect physiological conditions. Cells in a monolayer have unrestricted access to media components such as oxygen, nutrients, metabolites, and signaling molecules. On the other hand, *in vivo* tissue and cancer cells are affected differently by the presence of nutrients, oxygen, and metabolites due to the natural structure of their masses. It has been observed that 2D culture systems change the gene expression, interaction, topology, and biochemistry of cells. Furthermore, since it is a monoculture, it allows working with a single type of cell and does not allow the formation of the appropriate niche environment and tumor microenvironment required for tumor tissue (Kapałczyńska et al., 2018; Kucinska et al., 2021; Langhans, 2018; Verjans et al., 2018).

Due to all these disadvantages, 3D cell culture is widely used in drug studies and other important studies because it is more sensitive (Langhans, 2018).

3D Cell Culture

Advances in cell culture systems have allowed us to follow *in vitro* features that were previously only observed *in vivo.* A new generation of 3D cultures has been developed that can recapitulate multicellular type variability and morphogenetic behavioral diversity and will continue to evolve over the years (Chen, 2016). Our cells perform their activities in response to stimulation from a complex, 3-dimensional microenvironment (Burdick & Vunjak-Novakovic, 2009; Scott et al., 2010; Wan et al., 2005). 3D cell culture mimics tissue and organ-specific microstructure, allowing cells to grow in their normal physical shape, better cell-cell contact, and intercellular signaling networks. It makes it easier for them to complete their development and return to different complex structures (Saji Joseph et al., 2019).

The three-dimensional structure of cancer cells surrounded by neighboring cells and the ECM is critical for their metabolism and proliferation *in vivo.* ECM proteins and cells organize the morphology, function, and phenotype of surrounding cells. In conventional two-dimensional cell culture systems, these cell-matrix and cell-cell interactions are minimal or absent. Living and cancer cells often showed unnatural physiological responses to stimuli when removed from tissue or cultured in 2D cells. 3D cell culture models act as a transition zone between the structure in living tissue and 2D cell culture (Zhang et al., 2019).

In general, 3D cell culture techniques are classified as scaffold-based and non-scaffold-based systems due to the method of preparation (Pal, 2019; Saji Joseph et al., 2019).

Scaffold Based 3D Cell Culture

As with the ECM structure, it provides support for cells to proliferate, assemble, and migrate. In this cell culture method, cells are added to the matrix and the properties of the scaffold affect the cells. Preparing the environment for the cell to perform its natural function in the ECM is the main purpose of this scaffold. To some of the synthetic scaffolds, growth factors, hormones, and certain molecules can be added to increase cell proliferation or to support a specific cell phenotype. The design of the scaffold is based on the texture and properties of the cell. Cell compatibility and adhesion ability should be considered when determining factors such as porous structure, stiffness, and stability in the scaffold (Langhans, 2018). Hydrogels and solid-state scaffolds are two subbranches of this cell culture method.

Hydrogel Scaffolds

Hydrogel scaffolds of biological origin are water-swellable polymeric materials obtained by intermolecular (polymer network), interfibrillar and hydrogen bonds of monomers that make cross-link junctions (Justice et al., 2009; Worthington et al., 2015; Yan & Pochan, 2010). Although hydrogels exhibit solid-like material properties in their stationary state, the bulk of the volume with pores and voids between polymers is the hydrophilic polymer networks, facilitating the absorption and retention of large amounts of water. This organized system ensures that oxygen, nutrients, and drugs reach the proliferating cells, wastes are removed, and a suitable cell culture environment is formed. It is also considered a powerful method when applied for biomedical purposes (Deforest et al., 2010; Lee & Hubbell, 2013; Nii et al., 2013; Slaughter et al., 2009).

They can be produced from natural sources or synthetically to add new physical and biological properties. Hydrogels obtained from natural sources such as collagen, gelatin, fibrin, alginate, hyaluronic acid, laminin etc. are biocompatible with their high water content, low surface tension, soft consistency, and have natural adhesive properties, high cell viability, controlled proliferation, and differentiation, etc. enable the feature to be maintained. Collagen is the most widely used natural polymer (Ahmed et al., 2008; Allison & Grande-Allen, 2006; Badylak et al., 2012; Ehrbar et al., 2004; Orgel et al., 2014; Schmidt et al., 2008).

Synthetic hydrogels are also used in 3D scaffolds because they can mimic the biological properties of ECM. Due to their chemical and physical nature, they can be adjusted to achieve the desired hardness and porous structure. Polyacrylic acid, polyethylene glycol (PEG), polyvinyl alcohol, polyglycolic acid (PGA), and other non-natural polymers are the main synthetic materials used (Burdick & Prestwich, 2011; Langhans, 2018; Saji Joseph et al., 2019). The advantages of synthetic hydrogels are that they last longer, they have a high water absorption capacity, and they are relatively inexpensive. On the other hand, biological peptides need to be cross-linked with the scaffold to increase functionality, as there are no sticky parts found in the ECM (Gurski et al., 2017; Langhans, 2018).

Solid State Scaffolds

Solid scaffolds can be reproduced multiple times by controlling the location of cells *in vitro*. It can be conceived from dissimilar products such as glass, ceramics, metal, and polymer. Polymers are utilized to create scaffolds with different sizes, shapes, porosity, permeability, and stiffness adjustable (Duval et al., 2017a; Knight & Przyborski, 2015; Langhans, 2018).

Their controllability and reproducibility are their main advantages. The material used to construct the solid scaffold, its surface properties and permeability determine cell adhesion, growth, and behavior. Solid scaffolds are commercially available in sterile form. The material used to construct the solid scaffold, its surface properties and permeability determine cell adhesion, growth, and behavior. Solid scaffolds are commercially available in sterile form (Knight & Przyborski, 2015; Saji Joseph et al., 2019; Yamada & Cukierman, 2007).

Scaffold Free 3D Cell Culture

Spheroid Cultures

They are 3D cultures of clumps of cells that can be produced from a single cell type or a multicellular mixture of cells. It can be produced from immortalized cell lines, cells grown in primary cell culture, and cells derived from human tissue fragments. Low adhesion culture conditions encourage cells to clump together and stick together (Duval et al., 2017a; Pal, 2019). Commonly there are spheroids made from tumor cells, embryonic bodies, neuronal and hepatocyte cells.

3D spheroid model:

1. Imitating the natural structures of tissues,
2. To provide an ideal physiological cell-cell interaction,
3. Supporting the potential of cells to form their own ECM components and establishing good ECM interaction,
4. To perform the diffusion of growth factors and nutrients effectively,
5. It provides excellent compatibility for the removal of metabolic wastes (Breslin & O’Driscoll, 2013b; Fang & Eglen, 2017).

The size of the spheroids is basically based on the number of cells planted. Spheroids can grow similarly to target tissue if adequate oxygen and nutrient support is provided. Spheroids self-assemble and form clumps of cells (Yamada & Cukierman, 2007). It is an important advantage that they can be easily analyzed with a confocal microscope, an invert microscope, and a fluorescence microscope.

There Are Different Approaches to Spheroid Cultures

In the hanging drop method, there is no surface for cell attachment, and therefore the cells are collected spontaneously as spheroids. It was first developed in 1994 and formed the basis for scaffoldless models used to construct multicellular spheroids. In this technique, cells are cultured in a drop-shaped medium on the cover of the culture dish. Its cost, controllable spheroid size, and ability to co-culture various cell types are some of its many advantages. There is also the possibility of repeatability. It is difficult to change the medium.

The use of a low adhesion cell culture dish helps the cells to aggregate into a spheroidal shape. Low-adhesive containers are advantageous in that they are low-cost, reproducible, and prone to forming aggregates and spheroids that easily show 3D structure. These low-adhesion plates are coated with a special coating method that reduces surface adhesion. It has a higher volume capacity than the suspended droplet method (Duval et al., 2017b; Langhans, 2018; Saji Joseph et al., 2019).

Scaffold Free Organoid Cultures

In vitro 3D cell clusters that can self-organize, regenerate, and provide visualization of organ functionality are called organoids. They are often thought of as miniature versions of organs. Organoids can be manufactured from cell lines or primary tissues with appropriate cell attachment and survival support. Depending on how the organ buds develop, they are divided into tissue organoids and stem cell organoids. It is possible to make stem cell organoids from embryonic stem cells, primary stem cells, or induced pluripotent cells. There are different tissue organoid culture samples such as pancreas, liver, intestine, kidney, lung, retina, stomach, and thyroid (Achilli et al., 2012; Huh et al., 2011; Kunz-Schughart et al., 2004; Kuo et al., 2017; L. Li et al., 2016; Park et al., 2018; Souza et al., 2018). Organoids mimic the properties of real organs. There are several approaches to achieve it. The first approach is to produce organoids after cell culture is achieved in a monolayer on an ECM-coated surface and differentiation is ensured. The second is to ensure the differentiation of primary tissues by providing mechanical support. The third method is the production of organoids with hanging drops or containers with low adhesion surfaces (Breslin & O'Driscoll, 2013b; Fontoura et al., 2020; Kucinska et al., 2021; S. Li et al., 2021a, 2021b).

Conclusion

The 2D cell culture method has been one of the main methods for years in cancer research, drug experiments, scientific studies, and many more. Although it is an integral part of many scientific discoveries, it offers limited technology to understand the biology of organs. The major disadvantage of working with two-dimensional cell cultures is that it does not take into account that *in vivo* cells exist in a three-dimensional environment surrounded by other cells and ECM. Therefore, the results of such drug studies may not be accurate most of the time. Drugs found to be effective in two-dimensional cell cultures continue with animal studies before human trials. Unfortunately, most of these drugs fail at the clinical stage. In recent years, new drug discovery studies and tissue engineering have begun to use and develop 3D cell culture systems. 3D cell culture models provide more accurate and reliable data in drug research, as they improve cell-cell interactions and cell-ECM interactions. In this way, it is rapidly becoming a bridge between two-dimensional cell culture systems and animal models.

References

Achilli, T. M., Meyer, J., & Morgan, J. R. (2012). Advances in the formation, use and understanding of multi-cellular spheroids. *Expert Opin Biol Ther.*, 12(10), 1347-1360. https://doi.org/10.1517/14712598.2012.707181.

Ahmed, T. A. E., Dare, E. v., & Hincke, M. (2008). Fibrin: a versatile scaffold for tissue engineering applications. *Tissue Engineering. Part B, Reviews*, 14(2), 199-215. https://doi.org/10.1089/TEN.TEB.2007.0435.

Allison, D. D., & Grande-Allen, K. J. (2006). Review. Hyaluronan: a powerful tissue engineering tool. *Tissue Engineering*, 12(8), 2131-2140. https://doi.org/10.1089/TEN.2006.12.2131.

Badylak, S. F., Weiss, D. J., Caplan, A., & MacChiarini, P. (2012). Engineered whole organs and complex tissues. *The Lancet*, 379(9819), 943-952. https://doi.org/10.1016/S0140-6736(12)60073-7.

Breslin, S., & O'Driscoll, L. (2013a). Three-dimensional cell culture: the missing link in drug discovery. *Drug Discovery Today*, 18(5-6), 240-249. https://doi.org/10.1016/J.DRUDIS.2012.10.003.

Breslin, S., & O'Driscoll, L. (2013b). Three-dimensional cell culture: the missing link in drug discovery. *Drug Discovery Today*, 18(5-6), 240-249. https://doi.org/10.1016/J.DRUDIS.2012.10.003.

Burdick, J. A., & Prestwich, G. D. (2011). Hyaluronic acid hydrogels for biomedical applications. *Advanced Materials (Deerfield Beach, Fla.)*, 23(12). https://doi.org/10.1002/ADMA.201003963.

Burdick, J. A., & Vunjak-Novakovic, G. (2009). Engineered microenvironments for controlled stem cell differentiation. *Tissue Engineering. Part A*, 15(2), 205-219. https://doi.org/10.1089/TEN.TEA.2008.0131.

Chen, C. S. (2016). 3D biomimetic cultures: the next platform for cell biology. *Trends in Cell Biology*, 26(11), 798-800. https://doi.org/10.1016/J.TCB.2016.08.008.

Deforest, C. A., Sims, E. A., & Anseth, K. S. (2010). Peptide-functionalized click hydrogels with independently tunable mechanics and chemical functionality for 3D cell culture. *Chemistry of Materials: A Publication of the American Chemical Society*, 22(16), 4783-4790. https://doi.org/10.1021/CM101391Y.

Duval, K., Grover, H., Han, L. H., Mou, Y., Pegoraro, A. F., Fredberg, J., & Chen, Z. (2017a). Modeling physiological events in 2D vs. 3D cell culture. *Physiology (Bethesda, Md.)*, 32(4), 266-277. https://doi.org/10.1152/PHYSIOL.00036.2016.

Duval, K., Grover, H., Han, L. H., Mou, Y., Pegoraro, A. F., Fredberg, J., & Chen, Z. (2017b). Modeling physiological events in 2D vs. 3D cell culture. *Physiology*, 32(4), 266-277. https://doi.org/10.1152/PHYSIOL.00036.2016/ASSET/IMAGES/LARGE/PHY0041703840003.JPEG.

Edmondson, R., Broglie, J. J., Adcock, A. F., & Yang, L. (2014). Three-dimensional cell culture systems and their applications in drug discovery and cell-based biosensors. *Assay and Drug Development Technologies*, 12(4), 207-218. https://doi.org/10.1089/ADT.2014.573.

Ehrbar, M., Djonov, V. G., Schnell, C., Tschanz, S. A., Martiny-Baron, G., Schenk, U., Wood, J., Burri, P. H., Hubbell, J. A., & Zisch, A. H. (2004). Cell-demanded liberation of VEGF121 from fibrin implants induces local and controlled blood vessel growth. *Circulation Research*, 94(8), 1124-1132. https://doi.org/10.1161/01.RES.0000126411.29641.08.

Fang, Y., & Eglen, R. M. (2017). Three-dimensional cell cultures in drug discovery and development. *SLAS Discovery: Advancing Life Sciences R & D*, 22(5), 456-472. https://doi.org/10.1177/1087057117696795.

Fontoura, J. C., Viezzer, C., dos Santos, F. G., Ligabue, R. A., Weinlich, R., Puga, R. D., Antonow, D., Severino, P., & Bonorino, C. (2020). Comparison of 2D and 3D cell culture models for cell growth, gene expression and drug resistance. *Materials Science and Engineering: C*, 107, 110264. https://doi.org/10.1016/J.MSEC.2019.110264.

Gurski, L. A., Petrelli, N. J., Jia, X., & Farach-Carson, M. C. (2017). 3D matrices for anti-cancer drug testing and development. *Oncology Issues*, 25(1), 20-25. https://doi.org/10.1080/10463356.2010.11883480.

Harrison, R. G., Greenman, M. J., Mall, F. P., & Jackson, C. M. (1907). Observations of the living developing nerve fiber. *The Anatomical Record*, 1(5), 116-128. https://doi.org/10.1002/AR.1090010503.

Huh, D., Hamilton, G. A., & Ingber, D. E. (2011). From 3D cell culture to organs-on-chips. *Trends in Cell Biology*, 21(12), 745-754. https://doi.org/10.1016/J.TCB.2011.09.005.

Justice, B. A., Badr, N. A., & Felder, R. A. (2009). 3D cell culture opens new dimensions in cell-based assays. *Drug Discovery Today*, 14(1-2), 102-07. https://doi.org/10.1016/J.DRUDIS.2008.11.006.

Kapałczyńska, M., Kolenda, T., Przybyła, W., Zajączkowska, M., Teresiak, A., Filas, V., Ibbs, M., Bliźniak, R., Łuczewski, Ł., & Lamperska, K. (2018). 2D and 3D cell cultures – a comparison of different types of cancer cell cultures. *Archives of Medical Science: AMS*, 14(4), 910. https://doi.org/10.5114/AOMS.2016.63743.

Knight, E., & Przyborski, S. (2015). Advances in 3D cell culture technologies enabling tissue-like structures to be created *in vitro*. *Journal of Anatomy*, 227(6), 746-756. https://doi.org/10.1111/JOA.12257.

Kucinska, M., Plewinski, A., Szczolko, W., Kaczmarek, M., Goslinski, T., & Murias, M. (2021). Modeling the photodynamic effect in 2D versus 3D cell culture under normoxic and hypoxic conditions. *Free Radical Biology & Medicine*, 162, 309-326. https://doi.org/10.1016/J.FREERADBIOMED.2020.10.304.

Kunz-Schughart, L. A., Freyer, J. P., Hofstaedter, F., & Ebner, R. (2004). The use of 3-D cultures for high-throughput screening: The multicellular spheroid model. *Journal of Biomolecular Screening*, 9(4), 273-285. https://doi.org/10.1177/1087057104265040.

Kuo, C. te, Wang, J. Y., Lin, Y. F., Wo, A. M., Chen, B. P. C., & Lee, H. (2017). Three-dimensional spheroid culture targeting versatile tissue bioassays using a PDMS-based hanging drop array. *Scientific Reports 2017 7:1*, 7(1), 1-10. https://doi.org/10.1038/s41598-017-04718-1.

Langhans, S. A. (2018). Three-dimensional *in vitro* cell culture models in drug discovery and drug repositioning. *Frontiers in Pharmacology*, 9(JAN). https://doi.org/10.3389/FPHAR.2018.00006.

Lee, K., & Hubbell, J. A. (2013). Tissue, cell and engineering. *Current Opinion in Biotechnology*, 24(5), 827-829. https://doi.org/10.1016/J.COPBIO.2013.08.001.

Li, L., Zhou, Q., Voss, T. C., Quick, K. L., & LaBarbera, D. v. (2016). High-throughput imaging: Focusing in on drug discovery in 3D. *Methods*, 96, 97-102. https://doi.org/10.1016/J.YMETH.2015.11.013.

Li, S., Yang, K., Chen, X., Zhu, X., Zhou, H., Li, P., Chen, Y., Jiang, Y., Li, T., Qin, X., Yang, H., Wu, C., Ji, B., You, F., & Liu, Y. (2021a). Simultaneous 2D and 3D cell culture array for multicellular geometry, drug discovery and tumor microenvironment reconstruction. *Biofabrication*, 13(4), 045013. https://doi.org/10.1088/1758-5090/AC1EA8.

Li, S., Yang, K., Chen, X., Zhu, X., Zhou, H., Li, P., Chen, Y., Jiang, Y., Li, T., Qin, X., Yang, H., Wu, C., Ji, B., You, F., & Liu, Y. (2021b). Simultaneous 2D and 3D cell culture array for multicellular geometry, drug discovery and tumor microenvironment reconstruction. *Biofabrication*, 13(4). https://doi.org/10.1088/1758-5090/AC1EA8.

Nii, M., Lai, J. H., Keeney, M., Han, L. H., Behn, A., Imanbayev, G., & Yang, F. (2013). The effects of interactive mechanical and biochemical niche signaling on osteogenic differentiation of adipose-derived stem cells using combinatorial hydrogels. *Acta Biomaterialia*, 9(3), 5475-5483. https://doi.org/10.1016/J.ACTBIO.2012.11.002.

Orgel, J. P. R. O., Persikov, A. v., & Antipova, O. (2014). Variation in the helical structure of native collagen. *PloS One*, 9(2). https://doi.org/10.1371/JOURNAL.PONE.0089519.

Pal, R. (2019). *How are Organoids Different from Spheroids?* Retrieved February 24, 2022, from https://blog.crownbio.com/organoids-or-spheroids.

Park, J., Wetzel, I., Dréau, D., & Cho, H. (2018). 3D Miniaturization of Human Organs for Drug Discovery. *Advanced Healthcare Materials*, 7(2), 1700551. https://doi.org/10.1002/ADHM.201700551.

Saji Joseph, J., Tebogo Malindisa, S., & Ntwasa, M. (2019). Two-dimensional (2D) and three-dimensional (3D) cell culturing in drug discovery. *Cell Culture*. https://doi.org/10.5772/INTECHOPEN.81552.

Schmidt, J. J., Rowley, J., & Hyun, J. K. (2008). Hydrogels used for cell-based drug delivery. *Journal of Biomedical Materials Research. Part A*, 87(4), 1113-1122. https://doi.org/10.1002/JBM.A.32287.

Scott, E. A., Nichols, M. D., Kuntz-Willits, R., & Elbert, D. L. (2010). Modular scaffolds assembled around living cells using poly(ethylene glycol) microspheres with macroporation via a non-cytotoxic porogen. *Acta Biomaterialia*, 6(1), 29-38. https://doi.org/10.1016/J.ACTBIO.2009.07.009.

Slaughter, B. v., Khurshid, S. S., Fisher, O. Z., Khademhosseini, A., & Peppas, N. A. (2009). Hydrogels in regenerative medicine. *Advanced Materials (Deerfield Beach, Fla.)*, 21(32-33), 3307-3329. https://doi.org/10.1002/ADMA.200802106.

Souza, A. G., Silva, I. B. B., Campos-Fernandez, E., Barcelos, L. S., Souza, J. B., Marangoni, K., Goulart, L. R., & Alonso-Goulart, V. (2018). Comparative assay of 2D and 3D cell culture models: proliferation, gene expression and anticancer drug response. *Current Pharmaceutical Design*, 24(15), 1689-1694. https://doi.org/10.2174/1381612824666180404152304.

Verjans, E. T., Doijen, J., Luyten, W., Landuyt, B., & Schoofs, L. (2018). Three-dimensional cell culture models for anticancer drug screening: Worth the effort? *Journal of Cellular Physiology*, 233(4), 2993-3003. https://doi.org/10.1002/JCP.26052.

Wan, Y., Wang, Y., Liu, Z., Qu, X., Han, B., Bei, J., & Wang, S. (2005). Adhesion and proliferation of OCT-1 osteoblast-like cells on micro- and nano-scale topography structured poly(L-lactide). *Biomaterials*, 26(21), 4453-4459. https://doi.org/10.1016/J.BIOMATERIALS.2004.11.016.

Worthington, P., Pochan, D. J., & Langhans, S. A. (2015). Peptide hydrogels - versatile matrices for 3D cell culture in cancer medicine. *Frontiers in Oncology*, 5(APR). https://doi.org/10.3389/FONC.2015.00092.

Yamada, K. M., & Cukierman, E. (2007). Modeling tissue morphogenesis and cancer in 3D. *Cell*, 130(4), 601-610. https://doi.org/10.1016/J.CELL.2007.08.006.

Yan, C., & Pochan, D. J. (2010). Rheological properties of peptide-based hydrogels for biomedical and other applications. *Chemical Society Reviews*, 39(9), 3528-3540. https://doi.org/10.1039/B919449P.

Zhang, H., Zhang, J., Liu, Z., Xu, D., Guo, L., Liu, D., & Kong, M. G. (2019). Evaluation of the anticancer effects induced by cold atmospheric plasma in 2D and 3D cell-culture models. *Plasma Processes and Polymers*, 16(12), 1900072. https://doi.org/10.1002/PPAP.201900072.

Chapter 4

Bioprinters

Neziha Senem Arı[1,*], MD
and Elif Önder[2], MD
[1]Department of Histology and Embryology,
Kütahya Health Sciences University,
Kütahya, Turkey
[2]Department of Histology and Embryology,
Pamukkale University Medical School,
Denizli, Turkey

Abstract

Three-dimensional (3D) printers, which entered the world of science in the 1980s and are developing rapidly nowadays, offer easy solutions and product development opportunities in many sectors. The health sector is one of the areas in which 3D printing technologies are used. Thus, it is one of the most common methods in regenerative medicine and tissue engineering. Organ models are designed and attempted to be developed using living cells as a printing material with 3D printers utilized in the health field. Furthermore, 3D printers are used and developed in many fields, such as artificial tissue and organ printing, personalized medical devices, implant applications, production of various prostheses, pathogenesis studies of diseases, health education, and the pharmaceutical industry.

Keywords: 3D bioprinter, health, regenerative medicine, tissue engineering

* Corresponding Author's Email: drsenemari@yahoo.com.tr.

In: Bioprinting the Human
Editors: Soner Şahin and Kenan Demir
ISBN: 978-1-68507-993-2

Introduction

Three-dimensional (3D) printers are devices that have been developed as an alternative to 2D printers, which are mostly used nowadays, and that allow printing in three different axes by adding depth (Vanaei, 2021; Godoy, 2013). Although their working mechanism is similar to that of ink or laser-jet printers, they can produce for various sectors using different materials as a printing material. Since 3D printers were an expensive technology when they first emerged, it took time for them to become widespread. However, afterward, they found the opportunity to be tried in different areas with their prices reaching reasonable levels. Among the sectors in which bioprinters are used, there are many fields such as aerospace (Paletta, 2016), food (Godoi, 2016), textiles (Vanderploeg, 2017), construction (Kreiger, 2015), automotive industry (McCarthy, 2012), and health.

A three-dimensional model of the object to be printed is sent to the printer as a file using computer-aided design programs, scanners, and various radiological images in the health sector. After creating the first layer with the printer and the preferred printing material, the printing process is performed in thin layers one after the other (Giannatsis, 2009). In this way, many products can be produced in a short time or even within minutes, saving time and cost (Berman, 2012).

Although the beginning of studies in this field seems new, upon examining their historical development, it is observed that the studies date back to the 1980s. Hulls laid the foundations for 3D bioprinters in 1984 using stereolithography (SLA) technology, and the first 3D bioprinter company was established in 1986 (Hull, 1986). The established 3D Systems company produced the first 3D printer called SLA-250 in 1988 (Marciniec, 2004). Selective Laser Sintering (SLS), Fused Deposition Modeling (FDM), and Multi-jet Fusion (MJF) technologies have been discovered over time (Tagliaferri, 2019). Using SLS and FDM technologies, the first color prints were obtained, and thus 3D printers had the opportunity to enter the market.

Bioprinting Technology in Healthcare

Nowadays, a three-dimensional (3D) bioprinting method is one of the most common methods in the field of regenerative medicine and tissue engineering. Regenerative medicine is a science that examines the body's ability to self-renew and heal damaged cells, tissues, and organs under the effect of areas such as stem cell therapy, gene therapy, nanotechnology, and materials science (Gomes et al., 2017; Neagu, 2017; Matai et al., 2020). Tissue engineering is also one of the methods used to achieve these goals. Tissue engineering includes three basic elements such as cells selected in line with the study purpose; tissue-stimulating agents such as growth factors and signal molecules; structural scaffolds for the 3D culture medium. Tissue engineering with the basic elements it contains is an interdisciplinary application that fulfills the functions of damaged or lost tissues and aims to be sustainable (Langer and Vacanti, 1993).

The human body's ability to regenerate is limited. Current treatment options for repairing damaged tissues and organs are based on obtaining tissue from the same individual or transplanting it from cadavers. Organ and tissue transplantation is used to treat many severe conditions and diseases (Liu et al., 2021). According to data obtained from the Organ Procurement and Transplantation Network, 41,354 organ transplants were performed in the United States of America in 2021, with a 5.9% increase compared to 2020, and the annual total number exceeded 40,000 for the first time (Health Resources and Services Administration). There is a persistent shortage of patients on the waiting list for suitable tissue and organ transplantation (Rodríguez et al., 2021). With the increased shortage in this area, especially in recent years, the tendency to produce organs with biocompatible printers has increased. One of the main purposes of 3D bioprinters is to reduce this organ shortage.

Biofunctional inks are one of the main components of 3D printers. Three-dimensional printers print tissues and organs in a sterile environment using living cells as bioinks and make prints with cells in stacks to form a layered structure. The structure to be used as a bioink and filled into the cartridge, since it works with living cells, consists of cells produced and reproduced in the cell culture laboratory and a support material called a hydrogel, which will preserve and maintain the viability of these cells. Owing to the porous structure of this support material, cells communicate with each other to form tissue fragments. With advancing technology, organ models have started to be produced by printing different tissues at the same time (Mironov, 2009; Ozbolat, 2016). Moreover, the formation of organoids by bringing different cells and tissues together, establishing a mechanical and functional connection between them, and providing vascularization is among the promising areas (Marton, 2020).

To this end, Oberpenning et al., implanted bladders created with a 3D printer in dogs and monitored their functionality for up to 11 months (Oberpenning et al., 1999), and Hoerstrup et al., tested heart valves produced from autologous cells on sheep and goats and observed the normal functionality of their hearts for 5 months (Hoerstrup, 2000). In 2013, a bioresorbable material trachea was inserted into a newborn with tracheobronchomalacia (Bracci et al., 2013). The action potential was formed with synchronized contractions in the cardiac ventricular structure produced on a 3D printer with human cardiomyocytes, and wall thickening of up to 14% was observed during systole (Lee et al., 2019).

It is aimed that biological models and therapeutic products produced with a 3D bioprinting method in the field of health allow us to examine biology better, to replace structures lost for various reasons or removed by surgical intervention, by producing tissue and organ samples, and preserve their vitality. It is planned to examine these tissues and organs produced and their physiological functions in vitro, conduct pathogenesis research of diseases and cancers, drug studies, discover personalized cancer treatments, conduct studies in the field of toxicology, and use these developments in regenerative medicine studies for treatment (Lee and Sung, 2013; Yesil-Celiktas et al., 2018).

Since 2003, when 3D bioprinters started to be used, various implants such as hearing aids, special braces, brace implants, and spine and hip implants have been produced using this method (Banks, 2013). A pelvic implant was designed for a patient with pelvic chondrosarcoma (Gerrand, 2014). In a study evaluating 20 patients with acetabular fractures, models produced specifically for patients using radiological images of patients became a guide for surgeons during surgery (Hurson, 2007). Using this method, surgeries can be planned better before surgery. A study showed the design of wrist orthosis and stated that printers could be used in this area (Palousek, 2014). Another study observed implants made with a rapid prototyping design in 3 patients with different jaw problems for 1.5 years and detected no complications (Singare, 2005).

In terms of education, understandable models can be established for even the most difficult parts of human anatomy. In this way, the risk of harming patients will be reduced and time will be saved with these models in the process of learning how to perform a procedure in practical applications in the training of medical students (Torres Romero, 2019). A study examined two universities using educational materials obtained with 3D printers in their anatomy laboratories and stated that these materials eliminated ethical problems in the obtaining of bones and cadavers and were beneficial in terms of creating healthy and patient models in terms of diversity (Sugand, 2010; AbouHashem, 2015).

Another area in which 3D printers are used in the field of healthcare is the pharmaceutical industry. Studies in this area design models that ensure the preparation of personalized doses, especially for the elderly, elderly living in nursing homes, and for children and patients with organ failure for the ease of dose adjustment, and even for the simultaneous use of multiple drugs when necessary (Norman, 2017). The drug called Sprintam, which is used to treat epilepsy, is the first drug created with a bioprinter and has been approved by the Food and Drug Administration (FDA). In terms of ease of use, drugs that need to be taken in high doses can be taken as a single tablet, thus increasing the efficiency of drugs and ensuring the correct use of drugs (Dodziuk, 2016).

Conclusion

Studies on biofunctional inks continue worldwide, and the creation of the desired tissue and organ is promising for saving the lives of many more patients, whose treatment is possible only with tissue or organ transplantation, and for personalized designs.

The positive aspects of 3D bioprinters are that they can be used in various areas, they have high specificity in complex geometric shapes, and they are more advantageous in terms of time and cost compared to traditional methods. From this point of view, it is predicted that in the coming years, in addition to scientific and technological developments, 3D printers will become an indispensable part of daily life and will be widely used even at home (Berman, 2012).

References

AbouHashem, Y., Dayal, M., Savanah, S., & Štrkalj, G. (2015). The application of 3D printing in anatomy education. *Medical Education Online*, *20*(1), 29847.

Banks, J. (2013). Adding value in additive manufacturing: researchers in the United Kingdom and Europe look to 3D printing for customization. *IEEE pulse*, *4*(6), 22-26.

Berman, B. (2012). 3-D printing: The new industrial revolution. *Business Horizons*, *55*(2), 155-162.

Bracci, R., Maccaroni, E., & Cascinu, S. (2013). Bioresorbable airway splint created with a three-dimensional printer. *New England Journal of Medicine*, *368*(21), 2043-5.

Dodziuk, H. (2016). Applications of 3D printing in healthcare. *Polish Journal of Cardio-Thoracic Surgery, 13*(3), 283.

Gerrand, C. (2014). 3D Printing: a clinician's experience. *The Bulletin of the Royal College of Surgeons of England, 96*(7), 230-231.

Giannatsis, J., & Dedoussis, V. (2009). Additive fabrication technologies applied to medicine and health care: a review. *The International Journal of Advanced Manufacturing Technology, 40*(1), 116-127.

Godoi, F. C., Prakash, S., & Bhandari, B. R. (2016). 3d printing technologies applied for food design: Status and prospects. *Journal of Food Engineering, 179*, 44-54.

Godoy, P., Hewitt, N. J., Albrecht, U., Andersen, M. E., Ansari, N., Bhattacharya, S., ... & Hengstler, J. G. (2013). Recent advances in 2D and 3D in vitro systems using primary hepatocytes, alternative hepatocyte sources and non-parenchymal liver cells and their use in investigating mechanisms of hepatotoxicity, cell signaling and ADME. *Archives of Toxicology, 87*(8), 1315-1530.

Gomes, M. E., Rodrigues, M. T., Domingues, R. M., & Reis, R. L. (2017). Tissue engineering and regenerative medicine: new trends and directions—a year in review. *Tissue Engineering Part B: Reviews, 23*(3), 211-224.

Health Resources and Services Administration, Organ procurement and transplantation network. Available from: https://optn.transplant.hrsa.gov/data/,11 January 2022

Hoerstrup, S. P., Sodian, R., Daebritz, S., Wang, J., Bacha, E. A., Martin, D. P., & Mayer Jr, J. E. (2000). Functional living trileaflet heart valves grown in vitro. *Circulation, 02* (suppl_3), Iii-44.

Hull, C. W. (1986). *U.S. Patent No. 4,575,330*. Washington, DC: U.S. Patent and Trademark Office.

Hurson, C., Tansey, A., O'donnchadha, B., Nicholson, P., Rice, J., & McElwain, J. (2007). Rapid prototyping in the assessment, classification and preoperative planning of acetabular fractures. *Injury, 38*(10), 1158-1162.

Kreiger, M. A., MacAllister, B. A., Wilhoit, J. M., & Case, M. P. (2015, June). The current state of 3D printing for use in construction. In *The Proceedings of the 2015 Conference on Autonomous and Robotic Construction of Infrastructure. Ames. Iowa* (pp. 149-158).

Langer, R., & Vacanti, J. P. (1993). Tissue engineering. *Science, 260*(5110), 920-926.

Lee, A. R. H. A., Hudson, A. R., Shiwarski, D. J., Tashman, J. W., Hinton, T. J., Yerneni, S., & Feinberg, A. W. (2019). 3D bioprinting of collagen to rebuild components of the human heart. *Science, 365*(6452), 482-487.

Lee, J. B., & Sung, J. H. (2013). Organ-on-a-chip technology and microfluidic whole-body models for pharmacokinetic drug toxicity screening. *Biotechnology journal, 8*(11), 1258-1266.

Liu, N., Ye, X., Yao, B., Zhao, M., Wu, P., Liu, G., & Zhu, P. (2021). Advances in 3D bioprinting technology for cardiac tissue engineering and regeneration. *Bioactive Materials, 6*(5), 1388-1401.

Marciniec, A. D. A. M., & Miechowicz, S. Ł. A. W. O. M. I. R. (2004). Stereolitography-the choice for medical modelling. *Acta of Bioengineering and Biomechanics, 6*(1), 13-24.

Marton, R. M., & Paşca, S. P. (2020). Organoid and assembloid technologies for investigating cellular crosstalk in human brain development and disease. *Trends in Cell Biology*, *30*(2), 133-143.

Matai, I., Kaur, G., Seyedsalehi, A., McClinton, A., & Laurencin, C. T. (2020). Progress in 3D bioprinting technology for tissue/organ regenerative engineering. *Biomaterials*, *226*, 119536.

McCarthy, K. (2012). Improving rapid prototyping through the installment of 3D printers in automotive companies. *Honors Theses*, 2262.

Mironov, V., Visconti, R. P., Kasyanov, V., Forgacs, G., Drake, C. J., & Markwald, R. R. (2009). Organ printing: tissue spheroids as building blocks. *Biomaterials*, *30*(12), 2164-2174.

Neagu, A. (2017). Role of computer simulation to predict the outcome of 3D bio-printing. *Journal of 3D Printing in Medicine*, *1*(2), 103-121.

Norman, J., Madurawe, R. D., Moore, C. M., Khan, M. A., & Khairuzzaman, A. (2017). A new chapter in pharmaceutical manufacturing: 3D-printed drug products. *Advanced Drug Delivery Reviews*, *108*, 39-50.

Oberpenning, F., Meng, J., Yoo, J. J., & Atala, A. (1999). De novo reconstitution of a functional mammalian urinary bladder by tissue engineering. *Nature Biotechnology*, *17*(2), 149-155.

Ozbolat, I. T. (2016). *3D Bioprinting: Fundamentals, Principles and Applications*. Academic Press.

Paletta, N., Borrelli, R., Franchitti, S., Pirozzi, C., Piscitelli, F., Ferraiuolo, M., & Marini, M. (2016). *The Alm Applied to a Rocket Engine Injection Head–Development Plan and Material Characterization*. STO-MPAVT-264.

Palousek, D., Rosicky, J., Koutny, D., Stoklásek, P., & Navrat, T. (2014). Pilot study of the wrist orthosis design process. *Rapid Prototyping Journal*.

Rodríguez, D. A. S., Ramos-Murillo, A. I., & Godoy-Silva, R. D. (2021). Tissue engineering, 3D-bioprinting, morphogenesis modelling and simulation of bio-structures: relevance, underpinning biological principles and future trends. *Bio-Printing*, *24*, e00171.

Singare, S., Dichen, L., Bingheng, L., Zhenyu, G., & Yaxiong, L. (2005). Customized design and manufacturing of chin implant based on rapid prototyping. *Rapid Prototyping Journal*.

Sugand, K., Abrahams, P., & Khurana, A. (2010). The anatomy of anatomy: a review for its modernization. *Anatomical Sciences Education*, *3*(2), 83-93.

Tagliaferri, V., Trovalusci, F., Guarino, S., & Venettacci, S. (2019). Environmental and economic analysis of FDM, SLS and MJF additive manufacturing technologies. *Materials*, *12*(24), 4161.

Torres Romero, C. (2019). *3D Printed Prostheses and Organs*. Available from https://urn.fi/URN:NBN:fi:amk-201903243714.

Vanaei, S., Parizi, M. S., Salemizadehparizi, F., & Vanaei, H. R. (2021). An overview on materials and techniques in 3D bioprinting toward biomedical application. *Engineered Regeneration*, *2*, 1-18.

Vanderploeg, A., Lee, S. E., & Mamp, M. (2017). The application of 3D printing technology in the fashion industry. *International Journal of Fashion Design, Technology and Education, 10*(2), 170-179.

Wilson Jr, W. C., & Boland, T. (2003). Cell and organ printing 1: protein and cell printers. *The Anatomical Record Part A: Discoveries In Molecular, Cellular, and Evolutionary Biology, 272*(2), 491-496.

Yesil-Celiktas, O., Hassan, S., Miri, A. K., Maharjan, S., Al-kharboosh, R., Quiñones-Hinojosa, A., & Zhang, Y. S. (2018). Mimicking human pathophysiology in organ-on-chip devices. *Advanced Biosystems, 2*(10), 1800109.

Chapter 5

The Bioprinting Process

Aynura Agayeva*
Department of Histology and Embryology,
Uludağ University, Bursa, Turkey

Abstract

3D bioprinting is widely used in the creation of tissues and organs, such as vessels, hearts, skin, etc. It can also be used for pharmacokinetics, drug screening, etc. Since organs have a complex structure, various bioprinting methods are used.

Keywords: bioprinting process, 3D bioprinting technology, Inkjet-Based Bioprinting, Pressure-Assisted Bioprinting (PAB), Laser-Assisted Bioprinting (LAB), Stereolithography (STL)

Introduction

Bioprinting Process

The general 3D bioprinting process has three stages:

- Pre-bioprinting
- Bioprinting
- Post-bioprinting.

---

* Corresponding Author's Email: dr.a.agayeva@gmail.com.

In: Bioprinting the Human
Editors: Soner Şahin and Kenan Demir
ISBN: 978-1-68507-993-2

Prebioprinting

In preliminary bioprinting, the models used by the printer are formed in the first stage. Then the materials to be used in the process are selected. A tissue biopsy is performed to provide a biological model. At this stage, use magnetic resonance imaging (MRI) or computed tomography (CT). The images captured by these methods are remodeled to create 2D versions of these images. Then, the necessary cells for this process are allocated and reproduced. The cell mass is mixed with oxygen and various nutrients to maintain viability (Pereira et al., 2018).

Bioprinting

This is a printing process that forms a 3D structure using a biocinc. Biocinc is placed on a printer cartridge. He applies digital model-based material. The forming of biostructures is a bioink application to the frame in layers to create a 3D structure of tissue. This part of bioprinting is a complicated process, because it requires the formation of various types of cells depending on the type of organs and tissues to be created (Pereira et al., 2018).

Post-Bioprinting

Post-bioprinting is the final stage of bioprinting. It is necessary for the stabilization of the structure. Physical and chemical stimulations are required to maintain the structure and functioning of biological matter. These simulations allow for reorganizing and maintaining tissue growth. If this stage is crossed, there is a possibility of a violation of the mechanical structure of the material, and this will have a bad effect on the work of the material (Pereira et al., 2018).

3D Bioprinting Technology

Extrusion-Based Bioprinting

The most common method of printing non-biological 3D-structure is extrusion or microextrusion. It helps to study tissues and organs. Extrusion is the most commonly used method for the production of pharmaceutical dosage forms. This method uses printers that have a controlled temperature material delivery and processing system with a step, both of which can move on the x, y, and z axes. In addition, the system has a fiber optic light source to illuminate the application range to activate the photoinitiator (if necessary). Some of the micro-extrusion bioprinters also use more than one print head, which ensures the simultaneous issuance of several materials using the principle of extrusion-based bioprinting. Extrusion has two mechanisms for obtaining results; SSE (semi-solid extrusion) and 3D printing based on FDM (fused deposition modeling). A rotating screw mechanism or SSE with compressed air extrudes a continued flow of materials that are semi-solid through a nozzle, which is applied in layers to create a 3D structure. However, 3D bioprinting with fused deposition modeling (FDM) uses high temperatures to melt thermoplastic filaments. Which, in turn, after melting, are squeezed out through the nozzle layer by layer to create a 3D structure. 3D printers based on extrusion have two main components: positioning and the extrusion system. Both of these systems must work flawlessly to create a structure that is not only visually, but geometrically accurate (Placone et al., 2018; Sigaux et al., 2018; Papaioannou et al., 2019).

Examples of Extrusion-Based Bioprinting

The extrusion-based 3D bioprinting method is used in the biomedical, pharmaceutical and research sectors. This technology is usually used for the manufacture of frames that simulate the interfaces of tissues and is used in individual tissues. The technology is capable of producing models that mimic soft tissues and bone structures which provide an opportunity for possible implants (Placone et al., 2018).

Inkjet-Based Bioprinting

This technology has recently been used in the manufacture of three-dimensional (3D) structures and in medical applications. Cells, tissues, and some organ parts are used as bioinks and made available for culture applications. This technique has the potential to accelerate processes in tissue biofabrication. It can also be used in pharmaceutical distribution systems. It is widely used in research because it is a biologically applied technology in the field of tissue engineering (Algahtani and et al., 2018).

Inkjet-Based Bioprinting Techniques

Inkjet printing allows liquid droplets to be released onto the substrate. For thermal inkjet bioprinting, the thermal inkjet ink is electrically heated by the print head and creates pressure. The resulting pressure expels the droplets from the breast. Acoustic inkjet printing is done by placing a piezoelectric crystal inside the print head, which creates an acoustic wave. This breaks down the water into droplets. Due to the induction that occurs when a voltage is applied to this crystal, pressure is created. So he knows the droplets from the nozzle to the outlet. Both methods have their advantages and disadvantages, so the desired goal should be chosen correctly when making a decision (Li et al., 2016; Algahtani et al., 2018).

Examples of Inkjet-Based Bioprinting

It is widely used for the regeneration of skin and cartilage tissue. With this technique, biomaterials can be applied on tissue alone. This method can preserve the viability of cells and tissues. At the same time, stem cells can also be applied to the injury or damaged area. Recently, with the development of electrospinning technology, the possibility of creating it with all layers of cartilage tissue has been provided (Li et al., 2016; Algahtani et al., 2018).

Pressure-Assisted Bioprinting (PAB)

In pressure-assisted bioprinting, biomaterials are separated from the printer node by extrusion and form a 3D biological structure. Cells, proteins, hydrogels, collagen, chitosan, ceramic material solutions, and others can be used as biomaterials. This method can maintain cell viability by 40-80%. This disadvantage is due to the low speed of the printer. The fact that it can work at room temperature and homogeneous cells can be applied to the substrate shows the useful and advantageous side of this technology (Murphy and Atala, 2014).

Pressure-Assisted Bioprinting (PAB) Techniques

The pressure used in this technique is the pneumatic pressure generated by the coordinated, screw-style piston filament movement. By placing a fixed substrate, materials are laid in layers on it, and a 3D structure is obtained (Murphy and et al., 2014).

Examples of Pressure-Assisted Bioprinting (PAB)

Biomaterials in the form of a microscale nozzle or a continuous thread through the hole of a micro needle are extruded onto a fixed substrate. The most common biomaterials used are pastes, dispersions, and solutions. A 3D design is created by applying it in the form of a layer. The advantages of PAB technology include processing at room temperature, direct incorporation of cells, and uniform distribution of cells. Osteoblasts, mesenchymal stem cells, endothelial cells, and osteogenic progenitors can be bioprinted with this technique. With this method, oval calvarial defects can be repaired. There are also studies in which multipotent stromal cells in multicellular bioprinted structures differentiate into bone structures, as well as new blood vessel formations in progenitor endothelial cells. These studies show that the grafts formed with this technology can maintain their viability and mobility under in vivo conditions (Pereira et al., 2018; Papaioannou et al., 2019).

Laser-Assisted Bioprinting (LAB)

Traditionally, this technique was used only to transfer metals. Later, it was further developed, and today it has also started to be applied to biological materials such as cells, DNA, and peptides. A laser-assisted bioprinter consists of a pulsed laser beam, a focusing system, a ribbon with donor transport support, and a layer of biological material that has a receiving substrate facing the projector and is prepared in liquid solution. In this technique, biomaterials, cells, proteins, hydrogels, ceramic materials, and others are used. Bioprinters are able to maintain 95% cell viability. The speed level is moderate (Devillard et al., 2014).

The Principle of Laser Printing

It is based on the transfer of biomaterials to a solid surface one by one using a laser. Because the laser band is made up of a beam, liquid biomaterials evaporate and fall on the substrate in the form of droplets. Endothelial cells, fibroblast cells, and breast cancer cells of the pulmonary artery were obtained by laser-assisted bioprinting. By means of this technique, they have been able to create skin structures with appropriate cell density of co-layered tissues (Devillard et al., 2014).

Stereolithography (STL)

Stereolithography is a technique without free nozzles and is used to produce a 3D structure of biological and non-biological materials. The technique has a very high cost. During a process, a large number of biomaterials can be used. The material used is mainly a hydrogel. These hydrogels can form the desired target 3D structure by complying layer by layer. Stereolithography is a very fast method. The cell viability in the structure created by this technique is about 90% (Hong et al., 2021).

Stereolithography (STL) Techniques

Stereolithography technology, the principle of its work, is based on the solidification of a photosensitive liquid polymer. In this method, a digital micromirror is used which allows one to control the intensity of light. Photochemically liquid biomaterials or polymers are known to solidify and form layers that make up 3D tissue (Hong et al., 2021).

Examples of Stereolithography (STL)

It is known that human and animal tissues can be created with this method. This technique has also been tested on iDNA material, but it has not been found to be advantageous in terms of the fact that the UV rays used can cause DNA damage. It is believed that very advantageous results will be obtained if a light source is prepared for this that cannot damage DNA molecules in the future. However, a special light source can be prepared for use with DNA molecules (Placone et al., 2018; Hong et al., 2021).

Conclusion

Although 3D bioprinting is a promising method for a wide range of applications, it has been limited at the research stage and has not yet fully reflected itself in the clinic. But in the future, even more comprehensive techniques will be developed and used in the clinic.

References

Algahtani, M. S., Mohammed, A. A., & Ahmad, J. (2018). Extrusion-based 3D printing for pharmaceuticals: Contemporary research and applications. *Current Pharmaceutical Design*, 24(42), 4991-5008.

Devillard, R., Pagès E., Correa M. M., Kériquel V., Rémy M., Kalisky J., Ali M., Guillotin B., Guillemot F. (2014) *Cell Patterning by Lazer-Assisted Bioprinting,* PMID: 24439284. https://doi.org10.1016/B978-0-12-416742-1.00009-3.

Hong, Q., Lin L., Li Q., Jiang Z., Fang J., Wang B., Liu K., Wu Q., Huang C. (2021). *A Direct Slicing Technique for the 3D Printing of Implicitly Represented Medical Models* PMID: 34246156 https://doi.org/10.1016/j.compbiomed.2021.104534.

Li, J., Chen, M., Fan, X., & Zhou, H. (2016). Recent advances in bioprinting techniques: approaches, applications and future prospects. *Journal of Translational Medicine*, 14(1), 1-15.

Murphy, S. V., & Atala, A. (2014). 3D bioprinting of tissues and organs. *Nature Biotechnology*, 32(8), 773-785. https://doi.org/10.1038/nbt.2958.

Papaioannou, T. G., Manolesou, D., Dimakakos, E., Tsoucalas, G., Vavuranakis, M., & Tousoulis, D. (2019). 3D bioprinting methods and techniques: applications on artificial blood vessel fabrication. *Acta Cardiologica Sinica*, 35(3), 284. https://doi.org/10.6515/ACS.201905_35(3).20181115A.

Pereira, F. D. A. S., Parfenov V., Khesuani Y. D., Ovsianikov A., Mironov V. (2018). Commercial 3D bioprinters. In: Ovsianikov A., Yoo J., Mironov V. (eds) *3D Printing and Biofabrication. Reference Series in Biomedical Engineering*. Springer, Cham. https://doi.org/10.1007/978-3-319-45444-3_12.

Placone, J. K., & Engler, A. J. (2018). Recent advances in extrusion-based 3D printing for biomedical applications. *Advanced Healthcare Materials*, 7(8), 1701161 https://doi.org/10.1002/adhm.201701161.

Sigaux, N., Pourchet, L., Breton, P., Brosset, S., Louvrier, A., & Marquette, C. A. (2019). 3D Bioprinting: principles, fantasies and prospects. *Journal of Stomatology, Oral and Maxillofacial Surgery*, 120(2), 128-132. https://doi.org/10.1016/j.jormas.2018.12.014.

Chapter 6

Design of 3D-Printed Scaffolds

Sümeyra Ayan[1,6], Fatih Ciftci[3,4], Askican Hacioglu[5], Soner Sahin, MD[2] and Cem Bulent Ustundag[1,*]

[1]Department of Bioengineering,
Yildiz Technical University, Istanbul, Turkey
[2]School of Medicine,
Nisantasi University, Istanbul, Turkey
[3]Department of Biomedical Engineering,
Fatih Sultan Mehmet Vakif University,
Istanbul, Turkey
[4]Technology Transfer Office,
Fatih Sultan Mehmet Vakif University,
Istanbul, Turkey
[5]Department of Chemistry,
University of Helsinki, Helsinki, Finland
[6]Materials Institute,
Marmara Research Center, TÜBITAK,
Kocaeli, Turkey

Abstract

With the development of technological approaches in tissue engineering, treatment methods that are increasing day by day make life easier. The 3D printing method is frequently used in tissue engineering in the production of scaffolds, as it is cheap and provides ease of production. There are some parameters that should be considered in the design and production of these scaffolds to be used in tissue engineering. In this book

[*] Corresponding Author's Email: cbustun@yildiz.edu.tr.

In: Bioprinting the Human
Editors: Soner Şahin and Kenan Demir
ISBN: 978-1-68507-993-2

chapter, first of all, these parameters to be considered are specified. After that, information about 3D printers, produced scaffold, and characterization are given in this chapter.

Keywords: 3D printing, interconnectivity, natural and synthetic polymers

Introduction

Tissue engineering was an emerging field in the early 1990s that addressed the limitations of tissue grafting and alloplastic tissue repair, which involves transplanting biofactors such as cells, genes, and/or proteins into a porous degradable material known as a legacy structure (Hollister, 2005; Li et al., 2022). The components of tissue engineering are summarized in Figure 1. 3D structures provide numerous advantages from the chemistry of the arrangement and their porous nature in altering cellular activity through their architectural features that include pore and interconnection size. All these attributes can be used to tailor cell-material interfaces to tissue growth (Varma et al., 2020). For example, porous 3D scaffolds are relatively difficult to implant in cells because self-propagation is invalid and the initial density is low, especially in large structures. An example of new barriers that can be encountered when using scaffolding is that porous 3D scaffolding is relatively difficult to implant in cells because self-propagation is not uniform and the initial density is low, especially in large structures. In contrast, hydrogels can be generated in the existence of cells, leading to a more homogeneous dispersion and a higher charge density. However, rigid hydrogels with sufficient mechanical properties to perform rigid structures are often suboptimal in terms of cell migration and cell proliferation (Ovsianikov et al., 2018).

Conventional production methods were applied to fabricate porous 3D scaffolds, such as phase separation (Delgado-Rangel et al., 2020; do Amaral et al., 2022; Tu et al., 2021), solvent casting (Prasad et al., 2017; Sola et al., 2019), particulate leaching (Park et al., 2015; Sola et al., 2019), molding (Suárez-González et al., 2021), and foaming (Manavitehrani et al., 2019). However, all of these methods have significant problems. This means that we do not have enough control over the scaffold architecture, pore network and pore size, which makes 3D scaffolds inconsistent and inefficient. In order to overcome this mentioned problem, the researchers proposed the use of 3D printing techniques (also known as rapid prototyping, additive manufacturing or free forming) to create their own scaffolding with control, size and whole structure (An et al., 2015; Bahraminasab, 2020; Varma et al., 2020; Yan et al., 2018). The 3D printing, which has recently been increasingly used to make a variety of products, is not limited to prototyping (Kumar Mawandiya et al., 2021).

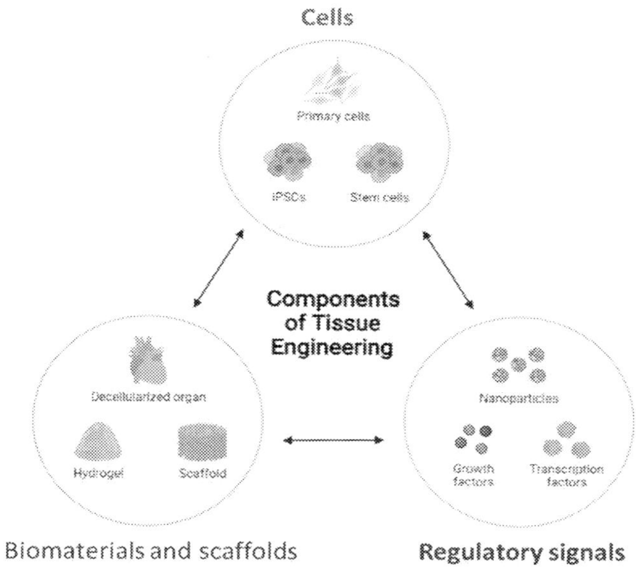

Figure 1. Components of tissue engineering, created with Biorender.com.

Biomaterials Applied for Tissue Engineering

Biomaterials are used in many fields (i.e., drug delivery, tissue engineering, etc.) due to their unique potential, such as good biocompatibility and bioactive properties (Han et al., 2022). The main biomaterials used in tissue manufacturing can be classified into four main components: synthetic polymers, natural polymers, composites, and decellularized matrices (Figure 2) (X. Liu et al., 2021). Because of the biocompatibility and nontoxicity of the scaffolds, the cells grown on the scaffolds must be able to proliferate and differentiate without interference to form a new matrix. The scaffold is considered an ideal scaffold for tissue engineering applications, because it can mimic the properties of ECM for complete and complete transformation (Eltom et al., 2019). Biomaterials are generally considered versatile, processable, and biologically functional. Although all biomaterials have been strictly tested, they are often classified as similar materials based on their composition. This adds to the complexity of selecting, testing and applying biomaterials, which in turn can lead to complex and erroneous procedures (Arjunan et al., 2022). Types of scaffolds for *in situ* tissue regeneration, as illustrated in Figure 3.

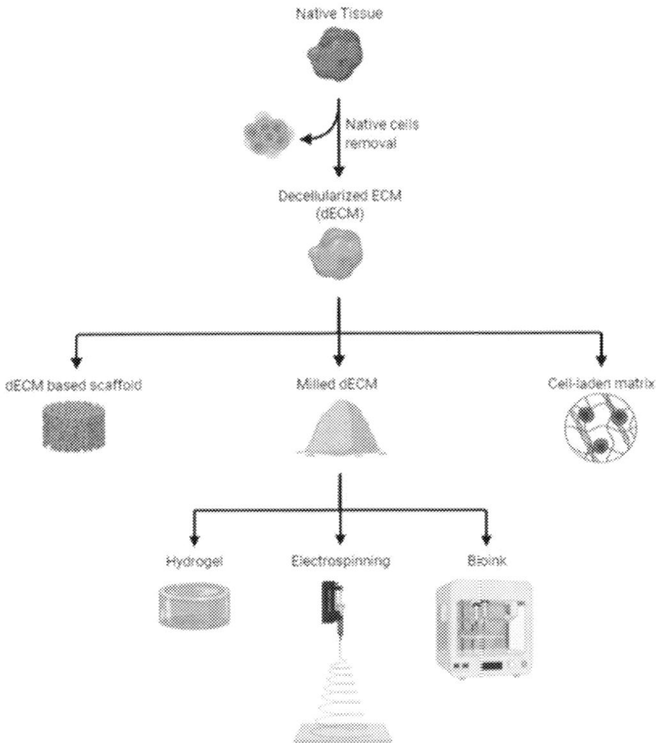

Figure 2. ECM-based biomaterials, created with Biorender.com.

Inks used in bioprinting that can be chosen to mimic the biological properties of the target tissue, called bioinks, are normally made from hydrogel-shaped biomaterials that contain therapeutic molecules. These scaffolds may contain cells of various origins and characteristics, such as autologous (umbilical cord blood mesenchymal stem cells (MSC)) or allogeneic (commonly used, such as neuronal or glial progenitors). MSCs are the cell type most tested, with beneficial effects on neighboring cells due to paracrine effects, making them excellent candidates for biomaterial incorporation (Ashammakhi et al., 2019; Oliveira et al., 2019; Zhou et al., 2019). Developed using bioinks as a filler and layer-by-layer deposition within a stenciled negative mold in the direct 3D printing process, 3D scaffolds are used to develop complex structures. These bioinks can be obtained from various natural resources (such as proteins, polysaccharides, etc.) and synthetic polymers (Sathish et al., 2022; Tarassoli et al., 2018).

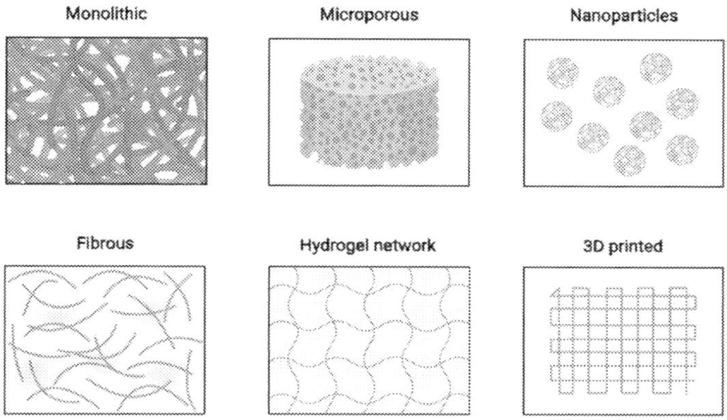

Figure 3. Scaffold types for *in situ* tissue regeneration, created with Biorender.com.

Natural Biomaterials

In comparison to synthetic devices, natural polymers, which are generally biocompatible, may also provide a superior microenvironment for cells. Natural polymers, on the other hand, are extremely difficult to 3D print (An et al., 2015). Polysaccharides are used in the production of biomaterials that can be easily adjusted and redesigned into the desired form using chemical modifications in their structure. Polysaccharides are readily available in nature and are cost-effective (Choudhury et al., 2021). The most studied polysaccharides to date are alginate (Falcone et al., 2022; Fu et al., 2022; Iglesias-Mejuto et al., 2021; Mallakpour et al., 2021), cellulose (Gauss et al., 2021; Nocheseda et al., 2021; Yang et al., 2020), chitosan and chitin (Pitrolino et al., 2022) in tissue engineering. Biocompatible and biodegradable alginate is an anionic biopolymer obtained from brown algae (*Phaeophyceae*). Alginate, which is easily formed in different stages, such as fiber, hydrogel, and sponge foam, is widely used in many industries (Chuysinuan et al., 2021). pH sensitive alginate polysaccharides are showing a steady increase for use in tissue engineering due to their attractive properties (Aguero et al., 2021).

Cellulose, which is the most abundant on earth in fiber form and has excellent mechanical properties, is used to produce 3D structures with 3D printing because it is cheap, light, durable, and recyclable (Abouzeid et al., 2020; Thibaut et al., 2019). The main structure of cellulose is a component of the main cell wall of green plants, oomycetes, and various species of algae (Muhammad Salman et al., 2021). In fact, until now, the possibility of using cellulose as a bulk material for 3D printing has not been fully explored. Additive manufacturing, net spraying, sheet lamination, and material extrusion using cellulose as the primary building block are reported as three categories of seven-layer manufacturing processes according to ASTM International (2012) (Dai et al., 2019; Thibaut et al., 2019).

Chitosan (CH) is a natural, biocompatible, nonallergic, and derived from the alkaline N-deacetylation of chitin found in the exoskeleton of crustaceans. If the number of N-acetyl-glucosamine units is high, the term chitin is used, and when the number of N-glucosamine units is higher, the term CH is used. CH can be broken down by ubiquitous enzymes in the human body and formed in various forms, and degraded oligomer products are capable of activating macrophages and promoting the synthesis of hyaluronic acid (Intini et al., 2018). Intini *et al.* fabric scaffolding with 3D printing without CH foil on the base is self-contained and integrated into two different 3D scaffolds, fibroblasts and keratinocytes with interfilament openings, using the Fuse Deposition Manufacturing (FDM) 3D printer. Furthermore, to get evidence for the properties of 3D scaffolds in order to develop tissue properties, they examined 3D scaffolds *in vivo* in terms of mimicking treatment characteristics using the diabetes-induced mouse wound healing model (Intini et al., 2018).

Synthetic Biomaterials

Poly (glycerol sebacate) (PGS) is a biodegradable, biocompatible, thermoset elastomer with good elasticity, soft response, and low inflammation prepared by polycondensation of glycerol and sebacic acid. These benefits make PGS the best candidate for tissue engineering, such as vascular remodeling, nerve induction, bone tissue engineering, and retinal detachment. However, the degradation of PGS *in vivo* is very rapid and the degradation of PGS products can produce local acids and store little water (Zhang et al., 2017).

Although PCL scaffolds have been widely used in agriculture, their material is rare and their water quality and low bioactivity limit their use in bone engineering. A good idea is to integrate biomaterials into PCL with bone tissue engineering biomaterials to increase their bioactivity and mechanical performance (Dai et al., 2022). There are many studies in the literature showing that different trace metal elements (i.e., calcium silicate, strontium, or magnesium) can contribute to tissue engineering applications. These studies confirm that these modifications promote bone regeneration. Lin et al., fabricated 3D scaffolds using strontium-doped calcium silicate in the center with magnesium-doped calcium silicate as the outer layer and PCL in order to develop the printability of the scaffolds. This enhanced magnesium and strontium architecture ensures a sustained release of ions to achieve the desired therapeutic targets, while preventing premature degradation of the scaffolds during immersion, although stem cell capacity has been shown to increase during the cultivation of these scaffolds. Additionally, hybrid scaffolds have been shown to enhance the expression of bone-related proteins, such as those that act on differentiated induction pathways containing TRPM7, PI3K/Akt, and WNT. The *in vivo* performance of the scaffold application was assessed using micro-CT (Lin et al., 2022).

Poly (ether ether ketone) (PEEK) semicrystalline thermoplastic polymers are widely used in areas such as the aerospace, chemical, and medical industries. Due to the advantages of excellent mechanical properties and radiolucency, PEEK is gradually being used in bone prostheses. However, the biological inertness of PEEK limits its osseointegration into surrounding natural bones, which is known to impede the long-term stability and clinical use of PEEK bone substitutes (Zheng et al., 2022).

Poly (vinyl alcohol) (PVA), one of the smart and stimuli-sensitive polymers, is used with increasing interest in 3D / 4D printing technologies in many applications including medicine and the environment. Reasons for the use of PVA in such areas include suitable flow capacity, sensitivity to stimuli, extrudability, biocompatibility, biodegradability, and cost effectiveness (Mallakpour et al., 2022).

Composites

Composite materials consisting of two or more components can be adapted to have a spatial arrangement to supply desired properties (Bahraminasab, 2020). Polyetherimide (PEI) is a compact high-performance biomaterial that meets the needs of orthopedic treatment. However, in order to receive better treatment, osteoinduction must be improved. Xu et al., The FDM technique was used to design orthogonal porous PEI scaffolds. Polydopamine (PDA) and

Arg-Gly-Asp (RGD) peptides were used for PEI/PDA/RGD scaffolds to simulate the extracellular matrix (ECM). The mechanical properties of the scaffold material are similar to bone tissue with good hydrophilicity and nontoxic properties. Extracellular bone matrix formation, adherence, calcium deposition and proliferation were reported to be higher in PEI/PDA/RGD scaffolds compared to other scaffolds (Xu et al., 2022).

In the study by Zheng et al., PEEK/HA scaffolds containing hydroxyapatite (HA) prepared in different weights were developed by the FFF technique to develop osseointegration with the master bone. The increased bioactivity and greater roughness of the HA-plus PEEK / HA scaffold results in greater bone volume and joint properties between bone and bone (Zheng et al., 2022).

In the study by Xu et al., fabricated a poly (ε-caprolactone) (PCL) microfiber scaffold with the actual direct writing device to prevent corneal fibrosis after injury, infused with rat tail collagen type I. They reported that the PCL/collagen scaffold imitated the stromal structure with properties similar to the natural cornea, and the PCL/collagen scaffold has good biological and mechanical properties. They also illustrated that the PCL/collagen scaffold decreased keratocyte differentiation (W. Xu et al., 2022). Zou et al., have recently developed a PCL and nano-hydroxyapatite (nHA) scaffold embedded with poly (lactic-co-glycolic acid) (PLGA) microspheres that enable controlled delivery. In their study, Icariin encapsulated with PLGA microspheres was embedded in the 3D-printed PCL/nHA scaffolds in order to simplify bone regeneration *in situ*. The scaffold has good mechanical performance thanks to nHA and they indicated that Icariin sustainably oscillates with the degradation mechanism. The icariin released from the 3D scaffold promoted osteogenic differentiation *in vitro* (MC3T3-E1) and *in vivo* (rat) (Zou et al., 2022). Therefore, in their study, Liu et al., the 3D printed alginate-gelatin hydrogel scaffold was coated with a thin layer of PCL to form the core/shell fiber scaffold. The PCL layer can reduce free radicals in the gel core. Next, PDA was coated on the prepared core/shell scaffold. Therefore, near-infrared (NIR) laser-triggered chemical release on demand (doxorubicin) has been reported in this system because of heat-induced sol-gel transfer from the central gel, such that tumor proliferation can be effectively reduced or eliminated *in vitro* and *in vivo*. They announced that they are planning a Gel/PCL/PDA core/shell scaffold as a platform to support wound healing. Especially for leukemia patients undergoing surgery, scaffolds can be implanted at the resection site to neither kill remaining cancer cells nor regenerate and repair tissue resulting from surgery (Liu et al., 2021).

The recording of the metal reinforcement phase and the production of composite scaffolding with this technology enables detailed geometry of the composite scaffolding with high resolution and accuracy. As such, it is a good way to develop biocompatibility, mechanical properties, and bioactivity of these scaffolds production process and structural properties of polymer-metal composite 3D porous scaffolding produced by 3D printing techniques (Zerankeshi et al., 2022). There are studies in the literature on self-expanding structures (scaffolds) to increase bone integration. However, although the improvement of scaffolds, the change in temperature and the disadvantage of bioactivity affect their chemical application. Zhang et al., adopted the NIR-sensitive and close-contact polyurethane image memory scaffold as the heat-sensitive matrix and photothermal and bioactive magnesium component designed by the 3D printer. As developed by Zhang et al., the scaffold composite has a homogeneous porous structure, greatly improving the mechanical properties and stable photothermal effect. Based on the results of the extrusion test and the finite element analysis, it was confirmed that the adhesion of polyurethane/4 wt% reinforced magnesium with the memory image was better compared to the medium without good memory. The osteopromotor function of scaffolds has been demonstrated by numerous *in vitro* and *in vivo* studies (Zhang et al., 2021).

The osteo-immunomodulatory responses of cellulose nanoparticles (CNPs) containing CH hydrogel scaffolds are not yet known. Patel et al., observed synergistic effects of silk fibroin and cellulose nanoparticles on the immunomodulatory behavior of CH biopolymer scaffolds. They fabricated CH/silk fibroin scaffolds reinforced with 3D-printed biodegradable cellulose nanoparticles (CH/SF/CNPs) and characterized them by different spectroscopic techniques. As a result, it has been reported that the produced hydrogel has a better rheological and recovery power than pure polymer hydrogels. They also observed enhanced bone regeneration *in vivo* with the Calvaria defect (Patel et al., 2022).

The strategy of integrating core/shell microspheres and core/shell microspheres with 3D printed scaffolds that provide bone morphogenetic protein-2 (BMP-2) was developed by Zhuang et al., for bone repair. The scaffold was printed with polycaprolactone (PCL) and then coated with PDA. The shells of the core/shell microspheres were electrosprayed with alginate, while the cores were fabricated from heparin-coated poly (lactic acid) (PLA) microparticles produced by a simple emulsion and heparin coating strategy. The hybrid system was interpreted in the rat critical-size bone defect model. They observed that core/shell microspheres tunable released BMP-2 and enhanced osteogenic performance *in vitro*, and their core/shell microspheres were subsequently successfully integrated into the scaffolds. They observed that the system combined with the resulting composite effectively promoted osteogenesis *in vitro* and *in vivo* (Zhuang et al., 2022). Sadeghianmaryan et al., have studied several combinations and drying of CH after the 3D printing. Therefore, they explained that the mechanical, physical, and mechanical components of CH scaffolds are designed for cartilage engineering and the appropriate concentration for CH printing alone should be low, the last one is 10%, but it shows low oxygen content. They also used alginate and nHA as impregnation solutions for printed scaffolds to create hybrid models to enhance the toxic properties of CH. The physical, mechanical and biological properties of the hybrid scaffolds were also characterized for their *in vitro* antibacterial properties and the potential for infection during the implantation of these scaffolds (Sadeghianmaryan et al., 2022). Although difficult to print, composites of collagen and CH are excellent materials for scaffolds. Suo et al., prepared collagen/CH bioinks with enhanced bonding through hydrogen bonding interactions and printing bonds. Rheological analysis showed that printed bioinks can change rapidly, strong shear thinning behavior with temperature 7-10°C, and cell viability analysis shows that cell strength increases and that it shows cell migration. CH can reduce print swelling, but the degradation rate increases with collagen ratio, while tensile strength and Young's modulus rate increase with CH ratio. In addition, scaffolds contain 2% (m/v) collagen and 2% (m/v) CH have a stimulating effect (Suo et al., 2021).

Design Parameters of 3D-Printed Scaffolds

Scaffold design requires control of chemistry, material properties, hardness, and surface topography, which significantly affect biological processes (Cubo-Mateo et al., 2020). To mimic natural texture, architectural features and the size of pores are important in the design (Gnanavel et al., 2022). The best way to improve bone scaffold geometry is to consider all variables (pore shape, pore size, pore ratio and pore connectivity) combined with various variables (material, permeability, and cell material response) to design clearly to achieve results (Bahraminasab, 2020).

Morphology/Architecture

With the principles of mechanics and geometry obtained, a suitable structure should have optimized surface properties for the attachment and migration of cells depending on the target tissue concerned. The external size and shape of the structure should also be considered (Hutmacher et al., 2014). Although the product is packaged in an image, there is no guarantee that the product will be 3D printable. Because the printing success of the vertical length also depends on the adhesion strength of the layers (An et al., 2015).

Porosity

Porous scaffolds are used as skin grafts and bone grafts to provide temporary support in injured areas. It is expected to have optimum size and porosity (important for adequate mechanical properties) to provide a suitable environment for tissue growth (Foroughi et al., 2022). Porosity is defined as the percentage of voids in a solid and is a material-independent morphological property. Surface permeability is important for tissue formation as it allows cell migration, growth, and vascularization, enhancing the interaction between plant biomaterials and tissues around the nose, and provides more than just safety to the critical junction (Karageorgiou et al., 2005).

Interconnectivity

Although the parameter of pore interconnectivity, known as the distance between two adjacent pores, at which cells spread to completely occupy a scaffold, affects cell behavior, there is insufficient information in the literature when compared with pore size, pore shape, and porosity (Varma et al., 2020). Porous meshes found in different materials have the main effects on material properties. Pore volume, pore size distribution, pore morphology, interconnections, and folds are quantitative pore parameters used to describe porous networks. Previous studies have shown that connections strongly influence transport properties (Fager et al., 2020).

Vascularization

Rapid vascularization of the substitute can ensure nutritional support, an interventional pathway, and channels for excretion for the immune system during the early stages of wound healing. That is why it is important to interpret the vascularization properties of dermal substitutes in the dermal reconstruction process (Chu et al., 2021). Although the macropore facilitates cell migration, nutrient, and oxygen diffusion as a key factor in scaffolds, it is not alone effective in directing the growth of vessels. It has been reported that scaffolds with microchannels that mimic the tubular structures of blood vessels can support invasion of blood vessels (Luo et al., 2022).

Fabrication of 3D Printing Scaffolds

The 3D printer raises bone formation with its cellular response and the porous structure to cell differentiation, cell adhesion, and cell proliferation (Gnanavel et al., 2022). The shape of the ultimate material comes from a CAD file (Hikmat et al., 2021; Mawandiya et al., 2021). Three methods are used for 3D printing techniques such as FDM (Jing et al., 2020; Szust et al., 2022), fused filament fabrication (FFF) (Roach et al., 2020), stereolithography (SLA) (Valizadeh et al., 2021), and direct jetting (DJ), photopolymer jetting (Behera et al., 2021; Dilag et al., 2019).

The FDM Technology

FDM technology is the most preferred 3D printer because it is easy, flexible in processing, easy to use, and material handling is able to be used as a continuous production machine. It is economically accessible and its raw material is commercially available for various applications. In FDM 3D printing, the printer head moves on the X and Y axes, and the up and down forces are generated by the bed (Z axis). The printhead has a heating element, which passes the filament through the heater and then keeps it in a semimolten state through the nozzle. At first, the printer provides the 2D model and then pushes the bed to raise the space between the bed and the headrest in order to adapt the next layer. Repeat the process layer by layer until you have a 3D model (Doshi et al., 2021; Garzon-Hernandez et al., 2020; Hikmat et al., 2021; Jing et al., 2020; Szust et al., 2022).

Fused Filament Fabrication (FFF)

If the feed material is a filament support, it is known as FFF. Generally, filaments are made from thermoplastics (e.g., PLA, acrylonitrile butadiene styrene, etc.) (Krishnanand et al., 2020). Capable of creating small to very large structures using a simple, wide variety of materials, compatible with a large library of mechanically sound materials (drones, satellites, antennas, mechanical enclosures), FFF 3D printing is one of the most widely used AM fabrication techniques (Roach et al., 2020).

Stereolithography (SLA)

Various 3D printing technologies, stereolithography (SLA) printing is a system that allows the manufacturation of solid objects at room temperature by polymerization of liquid resins under light irradiation, thereby reducing the risk of drug degradation, and drugs are able to be added into the resin in neither solution nor suspension before printing. Compared to 3D printing methods, SLA enables the precision fabrication of devices with a smooth surface finish, complex geometries, and superior feature resolution (Xiaoyan Xu et al., 2021). The SLA printing is suitable for large-scale application (Valizadeh et al., 2021).

Direct Jetting

Direct writing is a general term for additive manufacturing technologies that involve transferring, harmoniously depositing, and combining material onto a substrate in a predetermined pattern (Behera et al., 2021; Dilag et al., 2019). There are two ways to meet the demand for drip inkjet printing. The spraying can be carried out at room temperature or at room temperature. Steam radiators have a better solution. However, manufacturing seems to prefer the hot-spray process. Indeed, in most cases, rapid solidification occurs on high temperature surfaces. Also, since some hotspots follow the seal, it is advisable to use two different printing methods (Lee et al., 2004).

Photopolymer Jetting

The photopolymer jet (PolyJet) method uses inkjet printing to build objects, offering high resolution, allowing objects with smooth surfaces, and low polymerization shrinkage to be produced. The jet head drops photoresist through the nozzle to form layers of drops in a cross-sectional structure to form the final product, each layer being cured with UV light. In addition, the mechanical properties of 3D printed scaffolds can be improved by changing the polymer chemical structure, which expands the application scope. PolyJet is used in the manufacture of dental prostheses (Jacquet et al., 2018; Mai et al., 2017).

Characterization Methods of 3D Printing Scaffolds

Morphological Analysis

Morphological characterization of 3D printed scaffolds; SEM, TGA, powder X-ray diffraction analysis, static contact angle measurements, representative stress–strain curves of scaffolds under uniaxial compression load (Seyedsalehi et al., 2020).

Swelling Experiment

The swelling ratio of the printed scaffolds was measured by immersing the dry samples in PBS at 37 °C for varying time intervals. The swollen samples were weighed and then the swelling ratio was determined using Equation 1:

$$\textit{Swelling ratio (\%)} = (W_s - W_d / W_d) * 100 \qquad \textit{(Equation 1)}$$

where W_S is the weight in the swollen samples at a given time and W_d is the dry weight of the samples (Sadeghianmaryan et al., 2022).

Cytotoxicity Test

The scaffolds were placed at an average of 37°C, 60 rpm for 72 h, and the scaffold-free medium was filtered through a membrane filter. (C. G. Liu et al., 2018). In order to determine the cytotoxicity of 3D printing scaffolds for varying time intervals using the MTT assay (Intini et al., 2018).

Challenges in Optimization of 3D Printed Scaffolds

There are challenges in developing new material systems to use binder spraying for additively produced parts below 10 μm and to produce true 3D green parts. For reliable micro-AM, powder coatings, additives, and sealants should be 10 times lower than the main solution. This illustrates additional problems for the release of nanoparticle inks/slurries and bonding materials (Behera et al., 2021). The autologous graft is the gold standard for gingival and oral mucosal augmentation. Combined with smart polymers that can be printed with cells in a bespoke design, many natural 3D graft-like textures can be created. The 3D printing method is used for skin construction and vascular channel design (Nesic et al., 2020). Waste is a limitation of the SLS process when designing small structures, such as tissue engineering scaffolds. Incorporating small modifications into an SLS bed part solves this problem because the adapter can transmit movements from the SLS part bed to its own little bed (An et al., 2015).

Conclusion

The design of the scaffold requires the control of the material, the stiffness surface and the chemistry, which affect the biological process (Cubo-Mateo et al., 2020). The researchers proposed the use of 3D printing techniques in order to design their own scaffolding with control size and whole structure (An et al., 2015; Bahraminasab, 2020; Varma et al., 2020; Yan et al., 2018). Three methods used for 3D printing techniques are FDM, FFF, SLA, DJ, and photopolymer jetting. The 3D printing technique is critical in the production of functional scaffolds for tissue engineering and regenerative medicine, as it has the capacity to create complex parts (scaffolds, tissues or organs) with the use of different biomaterials (Pemmada et al., 2022). To date, photopolymerization of blood vessels has been investigated to create new pharmaceuticals, including 3D printing, oral dosage forms, hydrogels, multilayer polyps, microneedles, implants, hearing aids, and dental equipment, including the use of shape memory materials (Xu et al., 2021).

References

Abouzeid, R. E., Khiari, R., Salama, A., Diab, M., Beneventi, D., & Dufresne, A. (2020). In situ mineralization of nano-hydroxyapatite on bifunctional cellulose nanofiber/ polyvinyl alcohol/sodium alginate hydrogel using 3D printing. *International Journal of Biological Macromolecules, 160,* 538-547. doi: 10.1016/j.ijbio mac.2020.05.181.

Aguero, L., Alpdagtas, S., Ilhan, E., Zaldivar-Silva, D., & Gunduz, O. (2021). Functional role of crosslinking in alginate scaffold for drug delivery and tissue engineering: A review. *European Polymer Journal, 160,* 110807. doi: 10.1016/j.eurpolymj.2021. 110807.

An, J., Teoh, J. E. M., Suntornnond, R., & Chua, C. K. (2015). Design and 3D printing of scaffolds and tissues. *Engineering, 1*(2), 261-268. doi: 10.15302/J-ENG-2015061

Arjunan, A., Baroutaji, A., Praveen, A. S., Robinson, J., & Wang, C. (2022). Classification of biomaterial functionality. *Encyclopedia of Smart Materials*, 86-102. doi: 10.1016/ b978-0-12-815732-9.00027-9.

Ashammakhi, N., Ahadian, S., Xu, C., Montazerian, H., Ko, H., Nasiri, R., Barros, N., & Khademhosseini, A. (2019). Bioinks and bioprinting technologies to make heterogeneous and biomimetic tissue constructs. *Materials Today Bio.*, 1, 100008 doi: 10.10 16/j.mtbio.2019.100008.

Bahraminasab, M. (2020). Challenges on optimization of 3D-printed bone scaffolds. *BioMedical Engineering Online, 19,* 69. doi: 10.1186/s12938-020-00810-2.

Behera, D., & Cullinan, M. (2021). Current challenges and potential directions towards precision microscale additive manufacturing – Part I: Direct ink writing/jetting processes. *Precision Engineering, 68*(80), 197-205. doi: 10.1016/j.precisioneng.2020. 12.009.

Choudhury, P., Chawla, S., Agarwal, S., Singh, A., Nayak, A., Kumar, A., Maji, P. K., Goswami, C., & Goswami, L. (2021). Modified tamarind kernel polysaccharide-based matrix alters neuro-keratinocyte cross-talk and serves as a suitable scaffold for skin tissue engineering. *Materials Science and Engineering C., 121*:111779. doi: 10.1016/ j.msec.2020.111779.

Chu, B., He, J. mei, Wang, Z., Liu, L. lan, Li, X. li, Wu, C. X., Chen, C. sheng, & Tu, M. (2021). Proangiogenic peptide nanofiber hydrogel/3D printed scaffold for dermal regeneration. *Chemical Engineering Journal, 424,* 12846. doi: 10.1016/j.cej.2020.128 146.

Chuysinuan, P., Nooeaid, P., Thanyacharoen, T., Techasakul, S., Pavasant, P., & Kanjanamekanant, K. (2021). Injectable eggshell-derived hydroxyapatite-incorporated fibroin-alginate composite hydrogel for bone tissue engineering. *International Journal of Biological Macromolecules, 193(Part A),* 799-808. doi: 10.1016/j.ijbio mac.2021.10.132.

Cubo-Mateo, N., & Rodríguez-Lorenzo, L. M. (2020). Design of thermoplastic 3D-Printed scaffolds for bone tissue engineering: Influence of parameters of "hidden" importance in the physical properties of scaffolds. *Polymers, 12*(7), 1546. doi: 10.3390/polym12071546.

Dai, L., Cheng, T., Duan, C., Zhao, W., Zhang, W., Zou, X., Aspler, J., & Ni, Y. (2019). 3D printing using plant-derived cellulose and its derivatives: A review. *Carbohydrate Polymers, 203*, 71-86. doi: 10.1016/j.carbpol.2018.09.027.

Dai, T., Ma, J., Ni, S., Liu, C., Wang, Y., Wu, S., Liu, J., Weng, Y., Zhou, D., Jimenez-Franco, A., Zhao, H., & Zhao, X. (2022). Attapulgite-doped electrospun PCL scaffolds for enhanced bone regeneration in rat cranium defects. *Materials Science and Engineering: C*, 112656. doi: https://doi.org/10.1016/j.msec.2022.112656.

Delgado-Rangel, L. H., Huerta-Saquero, A., Eufracio-García, N., Meza-Villezcas, A., Mota-Morales, J. D., & González-Campos, J. B. (2020). Deep eutectic solvent-assisted phase separation in chitosan solutions for the production of 3D monoliths and films with tailored porosities. *International Journal of Biological Macromolecules, 164,* 4084-4094. doi: 10.1016/j.ijbiomac.2020.08.254.

Dilag, J., Chen, T., Li, S., & Bateman, S. A. (2019). Design and direct additive manufacturing of three-dimensional surface micro-structures using material jetting technologies. *Additive Manufacturing, 27,* 167-174. doi: 10.1016/j.addma.2019.01.009.

do Amaral, M. J., de Andrade Rosa, I., Andrade, S. A., Fang, X., Andrade, L. R., Costa, M. L., & Mermelstein, C. (2022). The perinuclear region concentrates disordered proteins with predicted phase separation distributed in a 3D network of cytoskeletal filaments and organelles. *Biochimica et Biophysica Acta (BBA) - Molecular Cell Research, 1869*(1), 119161. doi: https://doi.org/10.1016/j.bbamcr.2021.119161.

Doshi, M., Mahale, A., Kumar Singh, S., & Deshmukh, S. (2021). Printing parameters and materials affecting mechanical properties of FDM-3D printed Parts: Perspective and prospects. *Materials Today: Proceedings, 50*(5), 2269-2275. doi: 10.1016/j.matpr.2021.10.003.

Eltom, A., Zhong, G., & Muhammad, A. (2019). Scaffold techniques and designs in tissue engineering functions and purposes: a review. *Advances in Materials Science and Engineering, 2019*(4), 1-13. doi: 10.1155/2019/3429527.

Fager, C., Barman, S., Röding, M., Olsson, A., Lorén, N., von Corswant, C., Bolin, D., Rootzén, H., & Olsson, E. (2020). 3D high spatial resolution visualisation and quantification of interconnectivity in polymer films. *International Journal of Pharmaceutics, 587,* 119622. doi: 10.1016/j.ijpharm.2020.119622.

Falcone, G., Mazzei, P., Piccolo, A., Esposito, T., Mencherini, T., Aquino, R. P., Del Gaudio, P., & Russo, P. (2022). Advanced printable hydrogels from pre-crosslinked alginate as a new tool in semi solid extrusion 3D printing process. *Carbohydrate Polymers, 276,* 118746. doi: 10.1016/j.carbpol.2021.118746.

Foroughi, A. H., & Razavi, M. J. (2022). Shape optimization of orthopedic porous scaffolds to enhance mechanical performance. *Journal of the Mechanical Behavior of Biomedical Materials, 128,* 105098. doi: https://doi.org/10.1016/j.jmbbm.2022.105098.

Fu, Z., Ouyang, L., Xu, R., Yang, Y., & Sun, W. (2022). Responsive biomaterials for 3D bioprinting: A review. *Materials Today, 52,* 112-132. doi: https://doi.org/10.1016/j.mattod.2022.01.001.

Garzon-Hernandez, S., Arias, A., & Garcia-Gonzalez, D. (2020). A continuum constitutive model for FDM 3D printed thermoplastics. *Composites Part B: Engineering, 201,* 108373. doi: 10.1016/j.compositesb.2020.108373.

Gauss, C., Pickering, K. L., & Muthe, L. P. (2021). The use of cellulose in bio-derived formulations for 3D/4D printing: A review. *Composites Part C: Open Access, 4,* 100 113. doi: 10.1016/j.jcomc.2021.100113.

Gnanavel, S., & Kaavya, P. (2022). Design and development of novel 3D bone scaffold for implant application. *Materials Today: Proceedings.* doi: https://doi.org/10.1016/j.matpr.2021.12.580.

Han, X., Alu, A., Liu, H., Shi, Y., Wei, X., Cai, L., & Wei, Y. (2022). Biomaterial-assisted biotherapy: A brief review of biomaterials used in drug delivery, vaccine development, gene therapy, and stem cell therapy. *Bioactive Materials, 17,* 29-48. doi: https://doi.org/10.1016/j.bioactmat.2022.01.011.

Hikmat, M., Rostam, S., & Ahmed, Y. M. (2021). Investigation of tensile property-based Taguchi method of PLA parts fabricated by FDM 3D printing technology. *Results in Engineering, 11,* 100264. doi: 10.1016/j.rineng.2021.100264.

Hollister, S. J. (2005). Porous scaffold design for tissue engineering. *Nature Materials, 4*(7):518-24. doi: 10.1038/nmat1421.

Hutmacher, D. W., Woodfield, T. B. F., & Dalton, P. D. (2014). Scaffold design and fabrication. *Tissue Engineering: Second Edition, 2014*, 311-346. doi: 10.1016/B978-0-12-420145-3.00010-9.

Iglesias-Mejuto, A., & García-González, C. A. (2021). 3D-printed alginate-hydroxyapatite aerogel scaffolds for bone tissue engineering. *Materials Science and Engineering C., 131*, 112525 doi: 10.1016/j.msec.2021.112525.

Intini, C., Elviri, L., Cabral, J., Mros, S., Bergonzi, C., Bianchera, A., Flammini, L., Govoni, P., Barocelli, E., Bettini, R., & McConnell, M. (2018). 3D-printed chitosan-based scaffolds: An in vitro study of human skin cell growth and an in-vivo wound healing evaluation in experimental diabetes in rats. *Carbohydrate Polymers, 199,* 593-602. doi: 10.1016/j.carbpol.2018.07.057.

Jacquet, J. R., Ossant, F., Levassort, F., & Grégoire, J. M. (2018). 3-D-printed phantom fabricated by photopolymer jetting technology for high-frequency ultrasound imaging. *IEEE Transactions on Ultrasonics, Ferroelectrics, and Frequency Control.* doi: 10.1109/TUFFC.2018.2823545.

Jing, J., Chen, Y., Shi, S., Yang, L., & Lambin, P. (2020). Facile and scalable fabrication of highly thermal conductive polyethylene/graphene nanocomposites by combining solid-state shear milling and FDM 3D-printing aligning methods. *Chemical Engineering Journal, 402,* 126218. doi: 10.1016/j.cej.2020.126218.

Karageorgiou, V., & Kaplan, D. (2005). Porosity of 3D biomaterial scaffolds and osteogenesis. *Biomaterials, 26*(27):5474-91. doi: 10.1016/j.biomaterials.2005.02.002.

Krishnanand, Soni, S., & Taufik, M. (2020). Design and assembly of fused filament fabrication (FFF) 3D printers. *Materials Today: Proceedings, 46*(11), 5233-5241. doi: 10.1016/j.matpr.2020.08.627.

Kumar Mawandiya, B., Pancholi, K., Shah, D. B., & Joshi, S. J. (2021). Parametric study on process parameters of FDM 3D printer for thermoplastic materials. *Materials Today: Proceedings*. doi: https://doi.org/10.1016/j.matpr.2021.10.504.

Lee, D. H., & Derby, B. (2004). Preparation of PZT suspensions for direct ink jet printing. *Journal of the European Ceramic Society, 24*(6):1069-1072. doi: 10.1016/S0955-2219(03)00421-7.

Li, B., Wang, M., Liu, Y., Zhou, Y., Tang, L., You, P., & Deng, Y. (2022). Independent effects of structural optimization and resveratrol functionalization on extracellular matrix scaffolds for bone regeneration. *Colloids and Surfaces B: Biointerfaces, 212,* 112370. doi: https://doi.org/10.1016/j.colsurfb.2022.112370.

Lin, Y.-H., Lee, A. K.-X., Ho, C.-C., Fang, M.-J., Kuo, T.-Y., & Shie, M.-Y. (2022). The effects of a 3D-printed magnesium-/strontium-doped calcium silicate scaffold on regulation of bone regeneration via dual-stimulation of the AKT and WNT signaling pathways. *Materials Science and Engineering: C, 11,* 112660. doi: https://doi.org/10.1016/j.msec.2022.112660.

Liu, C. G., Zeng, Y. T., Kankala, R. K., Zhang, S. S., Chen, A. Z., & Wang, S. Bin. (2018). Characterization and preliminary biological evaluation of 3D-printed porous scaffolds for engineering bone tissues. *Materials, 11*(10): 1832. doi: 10.3390/ma11101832.

Liu, C., Wang, Z., Wei, X., Chen, B., & Luo, Y. (2021). 3D printed hydrogel/PCL core/shell fiber scaffolds with NIR-triggered drug release for cancer therapy and wound healing. *Acta Biomaterialia, 131:*314-325. doi: 10.1016/j.actbio.2021.07.011.

Liu, X., Wu, K., Gao, L., Wang, L., & Shi, X. (2021). Biomaterial strategies for the application of reproductive tissue engineering. *Bioactive Materials, 14* 86-96. doi: https://doi.org/10.1016/j.bioactmat.2021.11.023.

Luo, Y., Zhang, T., & Lin, X. (2022). 3D printed hydrogel scaffolds with macro pores and interconnected microchannel networks for tissue engineering vascularization. *Chemical Engineering Journal, 430,* 132926. doi: 10.1016/j.cej.2021.132926.

Mai, H. N., Lee, K. B., & Lee, D. H. (2017). Fit of interim crowns fabricated using photopolymer-jetting 3D printing. *Journal of Prosthetic Dentistry, 118*(2):208-21. doi: 10.1016/j.prosdent.2016.10.030.

Mallakpour, S., Azadi, E., & Hussain, C. M. (2021). State-of-the-art of 3D printing technology of alginate-based hydrogels—An emerging technique for industrial applications. *Advances in Colloid and Interface Science, 293,* 102436. doi: 10.1016/j.cis.2021.102436.

Mallakpour, S., Tabesh, F., & Hussain, C. M. (2022). A new trend of using poly(vinyl alcohol) in 3D and 4D printing technologies: Process and applications. *Advances in Colloid and Interface Science, 301*, 102605. doi: https://doi.org/10.1016/j.cis.2022.102605.

Manavitehrani, I., Le, T. Y. L., Daly, S., Wang, Y., Maitz, P. K., Schindeler, A., & Dehghani, F. (2019). Formation of porous biodegradable scaffolds based on poly(propylene carbonate) using gas foaming technology. *Materials Science and Engineering C., 96,* 824-830 doi: 10.1016/j.msec.2018.11.088.

Mohammadi Zerankeshi, M., Bakhshi, R., & Alizadeh, R. (2022). Polymer/metal composite 3D porous bone tissue engineering scaffolds fabricated by additive manufacturing techniques: A review. *Bioprinting, 25*, e00191. doi: https://doi.org/10.1016/j.bprint.2022.e00191.

Muhammad Salman, N., Ma, G., Ijaz, N., & Wang, L. (2021). Importance and potential of cellulosic materials and derivatives in extrusion-based 3D concrete printing (3DCP): Prospects and challenges. *Construction and Building Materials, 291,* 123281. doi: 10.1016/j.conbuildmat.2021.123281.

Nesic, D., Durual, S., Marger, L., Mekki, M., Sailer, I., & Scherrer, S. S. (2020). Could 3D printing be the future for oral soft tissue regeneration? *Bioprinting, 20,* e00100. doi: 10.1016/j.bprint.2020.e00100.

Nocheseda, C. J. C., Liza, F. P., Collera, A. K. M., Caldona, E. B., & Advincula, R. C. (2021). 3D printing of metals using biodegradable cellulose hydrogel inks. *Additive Manufacturing, 48(Part A),* 102380. doi: 10.1016/j.addma.2021.102380.

Oliveira, E. P., Malysz-Cymborska, I., Golubczyk, D., Kalkowski, L., Kwiatkowska, J., Reis, R. L., Oliveira, J. M., & Walczak, P. (2019). Advances in bioinks and in vivo imaging of biomaterials for CNS applications. *Acta Biomaterialia*, *95*:60-72. doi: 10.1016/j.actbio.2019.05.006.

Ovsianikov, A., Khademhosseini, A., & Mironov, V. (2018). The synergy of scaffold-based and scaffold-free tissue engineering strategies. *Trends in Biotechnology*, *36*(4):348-357. doi: 10.1016/j.tibtech.2018.01.005.

Park, H. J., Lee, O. J., Lee, M. C., Moon, B. M., Ju, H. W., Lee, J. min, Kim, J. H., Kim, D. W., & Park, C. H. (2015). Fabrication of 3D porous silk scaffolds by particulate (salt/sucrose) leaching for bone tissue reconstruction. *International Journal of Biological Macromolecules, 78,* 215-23. doi: 10.1016/j.ijbiomac.2015.03.064.

Patel, D. K., Dutta, S. D., Hexiu, J., Ganguly, K., & Lim, K.-T. (2022). 3D-printable chitosan/silk fibroin/cellulose nanoparticle scaffolds for bone regeneration via M2 macrophage polarization. *Carbohydrate Polymers*, *281*, 119077. doi: https://doi.org/10.1016/j.carbpol.2021.119077.

Pemmada, R., Telang, V. S., Dash, M., Charles Richard, J. L., Tandon, P., Ramakrishna, S., & Nanda, H. S. (2022). *Chapter 17 - 3D printing for functional tissue engineering* (C. P. Sharma, T. Chandy, V. Thomas, & F. G. B. T. T. E. Thankam (eds.); pp. 415–430). Academic Press. doi: https://doi.org/10.1016/B978-0-12-824064-9.00017-4.

Pitrolino, K. A., Felfel, R. M., Pellizzeri, L. M., MLaren, J., Popov, A. A., Sottile, V., Scotchford, C. A., Scammell, B. E., Roberts, G. A. F., & Grant, D. M. (2022). Development and in vitro assessment of a bi-layered chitosan-nano-hydroxyapatite osteochondral scaffold. *Carbohydrate Polymers*, *282*, 119126. doi: https://doi.org/10.1016/j.carbpol.2022.119126.

Prasad, A., Sankar, M. R., & Katiyar, V. (2017). State of art on solvent casting particulate leaching method for orthopedic scaffolds Fabrication. *Materials Today: Proceedings, 4*(2), 898-907. doi: 10.1016/j.matpr.2017.01.101.

Roach, D. J., Roberts, C., Wong, J., Kuang, X., Kovitz, J., Zhang, Q., Spence, T. G., & Qi, H. J. (2020). Surface modification of fused filament fabrication (FFF) 3D printed substrates by inkjet printing polyimide for printed electronics. *Additive Manufacturing, 36,* 101544. doi: 10.1016/j.addma.2020.101544.

Sadeghianmaryan, A., Naghieh, S., Yazdanpanah, Z., Sardroud, H. A., Sharma, N. K., Wilson, L. D., & Chen, X. (2022). Fabrication of chitosan/alginate/hydroxyapatite hybrid scaffolds using 3D printing and impregnating techniques for potential cartilage regeneration. *International Journal of Biological Macromolecules, 204,* 62-75. doi: https://doi.org/10.1016/j.ijbiomac.2022.01.201.

Sathish, P. B., Gayathri, S., Priyanka, J., Muthusamy, S., Narmadha, R., Krishnakumar, G. S., & Selvakumar, R. (2022). Tricomposite gelatin-carboxymethylcellulose-alginate bioink for direct and indirect 3D printing of human knee meniscal scaffold. *International Journal of Biological Macromolecules*, 195, 179-189.

Seyedsalehi, A., Daneshmandi, L., Barajaa, M., Riordan, J., & Laurencin, C. T. (2020). Fabrication and characterization of mechanically competent 3D printed poly-caprolactone-reduced graphene oxide scaffolds. *Scientific Reports, 10,* 22210. doi: 10.1038/s41598-020-78977-w.

Sola, A., Bertacchini, J., D'Avella, D., Anselmi, L., Maraldi, T., Marmiroli, S., & Messori, M. (2019). Development of solvent-casting particulate leaching (SCPL) polymer scaffolds as improved three-dimensional supports to mimic the bone marrow niche. *Materials Science and Engineering C., 96*, 153-165 doi: 10.1016/j.msec.2018.10.086.

Suárez-González, J., Magariños-Triviño, M., Díaz-Torres, E., Cáceres-Pérez, A. R., Santoveña-Estévez, A., & Fariña, J. B. (2021). Individualized orodispersible pediatric dosage forms obtained by molding and semi-solid extrusion by 3D printing: A comparative study for hydrochlorothiazide. *Journal of Drug Delivery Science and Technology, 66,* 102884. doi: 10.1016/j.jddst.2021.102884.

Suo, H., Zhang, J., Xu, M., & Wang, L. (2021). Low-temperature 3D printing of collagen and chitosan composite for tissue engineering. *Materials Science and Engineering C., 123*, 111963 doi: 10.1016/j.msec.2021.111963.

Szust, A., & Adamski, G. (2022). Using thermal annealing and salt remelting to increase tensile properties of 3D FDM prints. *Engineering Failure Analysis, 132*, 105932. doi: https://doi.org/10.1016/j.engfailanal.2021.105932.

Tarassoli, S. P., Jessop, Z. M., Kyle, S., & Whitaker, I. S. (2018). Candidate bioinks for 3D bioprinting soft tissue. *3D Bioprinting for Reconstructive Surgery: Techniques and Applications*, 2018, 145-172. doi: 10.1016/B978-0-08-101103-4.00026-0.

Thibaut, C., Denneulin, A., Rolland du Roscoat, S., Beneventi, D., Orgéas, L., & Chaussy, D. (2019). A fibrous cellulose paste formulation to manufacture structural parts using 3D printing by extrusion. *Carbohydrate Polymers*. doi: 10.1016/j.carbpol.2019.01.076.

Tu, Y., Ren, L. F., Lin, Y., Zhou, H. S., Shao, J., & He, Y. (2021). Fabrication of 3D hierarchical porous amidoxime-polyacrylonitrile spheres via nanoscale thermally induced phase separation with superhigh antimonate adsorption capacity. *Journal of Cleaner Production, 212,* 119-128. doi: 10.1016/j.jclepro.2021.127400.

Valizadeh, I., Al Aboud, A., Dörsam, E., & Weeger, O. (2021). Tailoring of functionally graded hyperelastic materials via grayscale mask stereolithography 3D printing. *Additive Manufacturing, 47,* 102108. doi: 10.1016/j.addma.2021.102108.

Varma, M. V., Kandasubramanian, B., & Ibrahim, S. M. (2020). 3D printed scaffolds for biomedical applications. *Materials Chemistry and Physics, 255,* 123642. doi: 10.1016/j.matchemphys.2020.123642.

Xu, W., Kong, B., Xie, H., Zhang, J., Liu, W., Liu, S., Zhang, Y., Yang, F., Xiao, J., Mi, S., Xiong, L., Zhang, M., & Jiang, F. (2022). PCL scaffold combined with rat tail collagen type I to reduce keratocyte differentiation and prevent corneal stroma fibrosis after injury. *Experimental Eye Research*, 108936. doi: https://doi.org/10.1016/j.exer.2022.108936.

Xu, Xiaoyan, Goyanes, A., Trenfield, S. J., Diaz-Gomez, L., Alvarez-Lorenzo, C., Gaisford, S., & Basit, A. W. (2021). Stereolithography (SLA) 3D printing of a bladder device for intravesical drug delivery. *Materials Science and Engineering C., 120*, 111773 doi: 10.1016/j.msec.2020.111773.

Xu, Xinyu, Wang, H., Zhang, S., Mei, X., Ying, B., Li, R., & Qin, Y. (2022). ECM-inspired 3D printed polyetherimide scaffold with Arg-Gly-Asp peptides for the improvement of bioactivity and osteogenic differentiation of osteoblasts. *Materials Today Communications*, *30*, 103166. doi: https://doi.org/10.1016/j.mtcomm.2022.103166.

Yan, Q., Dong, H., Su, J., Han, J., Song, B., Wei, Q., & Shi, Y. (2018). A review of 3D printing technology for medical applications. *Engineering, 4*(5), 729-742. doi: 10.1016/j.eng.2018.07.021.

Yang, J., An, X., Liu, L., Tang, S., Cao, H., Xu, Q., & Liu, H. (2020). Cellulose, hemicellulose, lignin, and their derivatives as multi-components of bio-based feedstocks for 3D printing. *Carbohydrate Polymers, 250,* 116881. doi: 10.1016/j.carbpol.2020.116881.

Zhang, X., Jia, C., Qiao, X., Liu, T., & Sun, K. (2017). Silk fibroin microfibers and chitosan modified poly (glycerol sebacate) composite scaffolds for skin tissue engineering. *Polymer Testing, 62,* 88-95. doi: 10.1016/j.polymertesting.2017.06.012.

Zhang, Y., Li, C., Zhang, W., Deng, J., Nie, Y., Du, X., Qin, L., & Lai, Y. (2021). 3D-printed NIR-responsive shape memory polyurethane/magnesium scaffolds with tight-contact for robust bone regeneration. *Bioactive Materials, 16,* 218-231. doi: https://doi.org/10.1016/j.bioactmat.2021.12.032.

Zheng, J., Zhao, H., Ouyang, Z., Zhou, X., Kang, J., Yang, C., Sun, C., Xiong, M., Fu, M., Jin, D., Wang, L., Li, D., & Li, Q. (2022). Additively-manufactured PEEK/HA porous scaffolds with excellent osteogenesis for bone tissue repairing. *Composites Part B: Engineering*, *232*, 109508. doi: https://doi.org/10.1016/j.compositesb.2021.109508.

Zhou, D., Chen, J., Liu, B., Zhang, X., Li, X., & Xu, T. (2019). Bioinks for jet-based bioprinting. *Bioprinting*, *16*, e00060. doi: 10.1016/j.bprint.2019.e00060.

Zhuang, W., Ye, G., Wu, J., Wang, L., Fang, G., Ye, Z., Lai, G., Qiu, X., & Sang, H. (2022). A 3D-printed bioactive polycaprolactone scaffold assembled with core/shell microspheres as a sustained BMP2-releasing system for bone repair. *Materials Science and Engineering: C*, 112619. doi: https://doi.org/10.1016/j.msec.2021.112619.

Zou, L., Hu, L., Pan, P., Tarafder, S., Du, M., Geng, Y., Xu, G., Chen, L., Chen, J., & Lee, C. H. (2022). Icariin-releasing 3D printed scaffold for bone regeneration. *Composites Part B: Engineering*, *232*, 109625. doi: https://doi.org/10.1016/j.compositesb.2022.109625.

Chapter 7

Bioprinting for Vascular and Vascularized Tissues

Rümeysa Göç[*], MD
Department of Histology and Embryology,
Cumhuriyet University, Sivas, Turkey

Abstract

Strategies to bypass blood vessels used to treat cardiovascular diseases have increased the trend toward synthetic grafts due to the scarcity of suitable grafts and the following reasons, such as thrombosis and infection. It enables vascular tissue grafts through 3D printing and in vivo integration, repair, and remodeling. Different scaffold-based additive manufacturing methods used in the production of vascular tissue, including bioprinting, 3D printing, bioinks, and electrospinning, are being tested. While attention was drawn to the functional and biomechanical requirements of the human vasculature, the efficiency of applying decellularization protocols to local vessels was evaluated. In addition, an interdisciplinary perspective should be provided for the development of vascular grafts by finding key elements and views of emerging technologies for successful clinical integration. Continuous advances in tissue engineering, decellularization, microscale additive manufacturing, and biofabrication are expected to be clinically viable and ready for use for small-scale applications in the coming years.

Keywords: bio-printing, bioink, vascular, 3D tissue vascularization

[*] Corresponding Author's Email: rgoc@cumhuriyet.edu.tr.

In: Bioprinting the Human
Editors: Soner Şahin and Kenan Demir
ISBN: 978-1-68507-993-2

Introduction

Autologous healthy blood vessel bypass surgery is a standard treatment for cardiovascular diseases. However, this treatment is limited to elderly patients and patients with vascular damage. (Veith et al., 1979) In addition, annually, millions of humans experience tissue or organ failure due to trauma, disease, or aging (organdonor.gov, n.d.). These needs have directed the development of technology toward the production of organs or vessels under in vivo conditions. The realization of the blood supply needs of the organs trying to be produced emphasized the importance of vascular structure.

The diffusion limit of oxygen from vessels is 100-200 μm. Therefore, the distance from the capillaries to the tissue cells is below this distance. Therefore, when the cell-containing tissue structure is implanted in the body, it triggers the damage recovery reaction and the inflammatory process, hypoxia, and angiogenic growth factor (GF) release. In addition, this stimulates spontaneous angiogenesis from surrounding tissues. However, Endothelial cells (ECs) have limited regeneration capacity; they can only cover 1-2 cm from the edges to the inside (Carmeliet & Jain, 2000). For this reason, prevascularization is mandatory to reduce the risk of cell necrosis in engineered tissues.

The vascular system carries oxygen and nutrients to tissues throughout the body (Krogh, 1922). Blood vessels are made up of cells and their extracellular matrix. (Marc, 1922) The plates consist of three layers, the tunica intima, the tunica media, and the tunica externa (adventitia). The tunica intima layer consists of the endothelium and the lamina propria. The tunica media layer consists of connective tissue formed by elastic and collagen fibers and circularly arranged smooth muscle cells (Clark & Glagov, 1985; Mirea et al., 2012). These muscle layers can cause vasoconstriction or vasodilation with the stimuli from the axons. The tunica externa is a connective tissue composed of collagen and elastic fibers. (Marc, 1922; Prince & Ahn, 2013) Nevertheless, in vivo implantation of extensive in vitro formed tissue or platform constructs yields if vascularization of the construct is not performed (Rouwkema & Khademhosseini, 2016). Capturing these features of the natural vasculature are the challenges of vascular graft development.

Freeze drying, phase inversion, and electrospinning (Ahn et al., 2015; Bourget et al., 2015; Diban et al., 2013; Mercado-Pagán et al., 2015; Qiu et al., 2009; Sekine et al., 2006; W. Wang et al., 2015) have tried to produce synthetic vascularized tissue structures and vascular grafts (Tremblay et al., 2005; Zhang et al., 2015). However, it suffers from imperfect command over the internal system and general geometry shapes of three-dimensional (3D) structures (Yang et al., 2002). On the other hand, additive manufacturing (AM) techniques to regulate the biomimetic complexity of engineered systems offer great flexibility in their automated production (Feng & Ye, 2011; Melchels et al., 2012). Thanks to AM, approaches with autologous cell sources, antithrombogenic biomaterials, and modern medical imaging techniques are opening new horizons for rapid tissue regeneration and the production of grafts in vivo (Paulsen & Miller, 2015; Visconti et al., 2010).

Techniques for providing vascularization of tissue structures that do not have a blood supply are as follows:

1. Designing porous scaffolds that allow the formation of new vessels after implantation
2. External delivery of angiogenic growth factors, cells, or cytokines to implanted materials
3. The surface immobilizes complete proteins or regulates peptide sequences to enable angiogenesis in engineered tissues within the body (Druecke et al., 2004; Lovett et al., 2009).

The prevascularization process in tissues produced in laboratories depends on endothelial cells (ECs) to self-organize and form vascular networks (Freiman et al., 2016; Santos et al., 2008; Stahl et al., 2014). However, bioprinting of vascularized tissues or organs requires optimization of the different components of the bioink used. Among other methods, attempts have been made to preserve the tissue skeleton by decellularizing the natural vasculature (Cross & Claesson-Welsh, 2001) or human placenta (Carmeliet, 2004). In one study, agarose was used in 3D printing while making a double-layered vascular tube placed horizontally on an assembly of fibroblast and smooth muscle cells (Carmeliet, 2004). As with other techniques, bioprinting efforts using hydrogels and synthetic polymers have also been tested on multilayer vessel walls (Hoch et al., 2014; Skardal et al., 2010c; Skardal et al., 2010a; Skardal et al., 2010b). One study (Wu & Ringeisen, 2010) demonstrated the onset of cell-cell connections and luminal-like formation between endothelial and smooth muscle cells closely pressed against each other. Therefore, designing the tunica intima, tunica media, and tunica externa considering vascular histological features will require consideration for next-generation vascular prostheses. The number and thickness of the layers vary according to the physiological task performed by the vessels. While the capillaries are 9 μm in diameter, they are surrounded by only a single layer of EC, allowing oxygen and nutrients to diffuse quickly and efficiently. While the diameter range of the arteries is 0.6-16 mm, their walls are thick and flexible due to high pressure.

On the other hand, vessels with a diameter of 1-15 mm maintain hypotension, so they are easily deformed and have a thin wall that lacks the apparent structural community of the arteries (Wu & Ringeisen, 2010). Intercalarily, the extracellular matrix (ECM), which is the connective tissue of the vessel, plays a vital role in the natural mechanical structure (Wu & Ringeisen, 2010). Compressibility, tensile stiffness, viscoelasticity, and elasticity properties are crucial for the correct functioning of the tissue. In the tunica adventitia layers of human coronary arteries, there is a longitudinal tension of 1300 ± 692 kPa and a circumferential pressure of 1430 ± 604 kPa. While tensile stress mainly occurs by type I and III collagen, proteoglycans provide compressibility (Wu & Ringeisen, 2010). While the viscoelasticity is together with collagen and elastin, elastin fibers assume the elasticity.

To design bioprinted vascular networks, it is necessary to know the vasculogenesis and angiogenesis. Vasculogenesis is the construction of new blood vessels during embryogenesis. In vasculogenesis, angioblasts, embryonic vascular precursor stem cells, relocate from the splenic mesoderm to form blood islets. These structures are then differentiated into endothelial progenitor cells (EPCs). Finally, EPCs are arranged to assemble in tubular structures and form primal microcapillaries. In adults, we see vasculogenesis in tumor growth or tissue healing (Wu & Ringeisen, 2010).

Angiogenesis is the building of new vessels by branching from preexisting vascular networks. In the absence of oxygen and nutrients developing in tissues, the ECs are separated from their places, and their branching is cauterized to reach the hypoxic region (Carmeliet, 2000; Rouwkema & Khademhosseini, 2016). During angiogenesis, growth factors play a decisive role. Its main components are the essential fibroblast growth factor (bFGF), Vascular endothelial growth factor (VEGF), and platelet-derived growth factor (PDGF or CD31) (Cross & Claesson-Welsh, 2001). bFGF promotes migration, proliferation, and differentiation of ECs, while VEGF is created by numerous cells and is a chemoattractive and mighty mitogen for ECs. In addition, PDGFs promote remodeling and maturation.

Bioprinting Materials

Bioprinting is an additive manufacturing technique of hydrogel-containing bioink material to encapsulate aggregates or cells. Bioinks can be constructed from synthetic, natural or biomaterials (Gungor-Ozkerim et al., 2018). These bioinks must comply with the biological and mechanical effects of the tissue and meet the bioprinting modalities. In addition, cross-linking in the bioprinting process should allow the preservation of the structure and support cell viability and functionality. A bioink must have a specific gelling and viscosity capacity and a certain shear rate to be processed (Jungst et al., 2016). In addition, after the bioprinting process is finished, the bioink is protected. The faster the Bioink undergoes gelation and solidification, the higher the solubility.

Naturally Derived Bioinks

Collagen, fibrin, hyaluronic acid, gelatin, agarose, and alginate are naturally derived bioinks. Since these structures are already components of the ECM, they have an inherent advantage (Gomes et al., 2012). However, since they do not have high mechanical belongings, cells have a weak 3D computerized background. Therefore, it is combined with other natural polymers such as agarose, collagen, and fibrinogen to improve cell adhesion and proliferation (Kreimendahl et al., 2017). Collagen-agarose hydrogels showed greater storage capacity compared to individual use. While no degradation was observed in the blends, fibrin-agarose hydrogels showed greater water uptake than collagen-agarose hydrogels. However, cell migration enhanced capillary formation and shape stabilization was honored with the coculture of ECs and fibroblasts in collagen-agarose hydrogels compared to fibrinogen-collagen hydrogels (Norotte et al., 2009). After culture of alginates with HUVECs, a monolayer endothelium with permeability and remodeling properties was formed. Collagen has been used as a bio-paper in combination with other bio-inks. Biopapers are flat biomimetic scaffolds produced by molding (Pirlo et al., 2012) or electrospinning (Catros et al., 2012), creating 3D cell printing (Brandt, 2017).

Synthetic Bioinks

Synthetic bioinks are chemically modifiable as well as have high reproducibility and usability. In this way, they can be customized and versatile for specific purposes. Cells do not have adhesion sites, although their mechanical properties are tunable. Pluronic ® is a widely used polyoxyethylene–polyoxypropylene–polyoxyethylene (PEO–PPO–PEO) amphiphilic triblock copolymer (or poloxamer) (Bohorquez et al., 1999). Carbohydrate glasses for bioprinting can also be perfused and templated, covered by biocompatible cell-loaded hydrogels to form cylindrical canal networks. Carbohydrate glasses are mixed with dextrans to keep them intact even at higher temperatures. Additionally, it is coated with poly(D-lactide-co-glycolide) (PDLGA) upon extrusion to prevent cell osmotic damage. That allows forming channels with other surrounding biomaterials such as agarose, alginate, PEG, fibrin, and Matrigel (Miller et al., 2012).

Cells, Co-Culture Systems, and Spheroids

Blood vessels are composed of three different cell types: endothelial cells (EC), smooth muscle cells (SMC), and fibroblasts. ECs are separated from the arteries or veins of different tissues, with the most familiar source being the umbilical cord vessel (HUVEC) (Gao et al., 2018; V. K. Lee et al., 2014). (iPSCs) (Rosa et al., 2019) and endothelial colony-forming cells (ECFCs) (Paschalaki & Randi, 2018) are also preferred among stem cell sources. Conversely, for ECFCs, they are usually cells sequestered from peripheral blood or cord blood (Paschalaki & Randi, 2018).

SMCs in blood vessels are close to ECs and are located in the interlayer (G. Wang et al., 2015). SMCs provide the high plasticity required for ECM synthesis and cell proliferation, although vessel contraction is their primary task (Novosel et al., 2011). In one study, vascular SMCs were bioprinted utilizing an inherently emanated hydrogel as transport (Tijore et al., 2018). Aligned SMCs persist along the microchannels to maintain the contraction-elongation phenotype. α-smooth muscle actin (α-SMA) and smooth muscle myosin heavy chain (SM-MHC) gene markers were also observed in the produced vessels after seven days of culture. SMCs transformed from iPSCs, or endothelial mesenchymal are promising sources for bioprinting (Frid et al., 2002; Maguire et al., 2017). However, it is unclear whether transdifferentiated SMCs can maintain contractility and exhibit plasticity. Fibroblasts are transdifferentiated from MSCs located in the tunica adventitia and are involved in the synthesizing of ECM molecules after activation. In vascular bioprinting, Gao et al. were able to print mouse fibroblasts in alginate, which reached viability of 92.9 ± 2.4% after 24 hours of culture.

The culture of fibroblasts and HUVECs was assayed in a thrombosis model on a chip by 3D bioprinting. CD31 staining confirmed that HUVECs are located along the microchannel, even in forked channels. In endothelial damaged modeling, it was observed that fibroblasts accumulated a high amount of collagen. MSCs, multipotent stem cells used in cocultures, have improved angiogenesis and regulated hemopoietic stem cell function. After bioprinting, MSCs have been shown to form endothelial-like cells and maintain cell viability. In addition, MSCs are involved in cardiac regeneration and remodeling. Therefore, it was bioprinted with MSCs and HUVECs using the laser bioprinting technique on the cardiac patch. MSCs increased factor and ECM secretion in cocultures, while HUVECs improved vascular differentiation and cell survival. Cell clusters (spheroids) are used in bioprinting. Tissue spheroids or microtissues can be combined as constructing obstructions to form macro tissues or organs (McAnulty, 2007). The tissues produced are structurally and functionally very similar to the natural tissue environment and are used in matrix remodeling, angiogenesis, and drug screening studies (Lin & Chang, 2008). It forms stable spheroids in agarose microwells by adipose tissue-derived mesenchymal stem cells (ADSCs) or fibroblasts, or a combination of both. The addition of ADSCs produced larger-scale ECM production, a capillary-like network, and spheroids with uniform HUVEC distribution were printed with an airflow-assisted 3D bioprinter (Zhao et al., 2018).

Tissue Vascularization

While spontaneous vascularization may be acceptable when targeting thin tissues such as skin or other avascular tissues such as cartilage, difficulties appear in more significant imperfections in which oxygen and nutrient diffusion gradients are measured (Malda et al., 2004). This is essential for tissues such as bone, where critical-sized defects are often several centimeters long (Bose et al., 2012; Santos & Reis, 2010). Therefore, studies have been carried out to integrate the vascular network in bioimprinted tissues, particularly in the thyroid (Bulanova et al., 2017), kidney, cardiac tissue (K.

Wang et al., 2019), muscle (Choi et al., 2019), liver (J. W. Lee et al., 2016), and bone (Byambaa et al., 2017; Cui et al., 2016).

In order to simulate the structure of bone, a biphasic platform surrounded by a rigid mineral core and weak matrix was developed, combining stereolithography (SLA) and fused deposition modeling (FDM). The prominent part, which will form the mineral core by FDM printing, was produced with biocompatible polylactic acid (PLA). Parenchymal and nonparenchymal stem cells were cultured with angiogenesis in bioprinted form for the liver (J. W. Lee et al., 2016). Human lung fibroblasts (HLFs), HUVECs, and hepatocytes (HCs) were cocultured in collagen bioink in a PCL framework. This coculture system provided a 3D culture medium that increased the functionality and viability of HCs by interacting with the ECM. In a recently completed study, bioprinting was used to fabricate produced kidneys and explore the selective renal re-absorption of glucose and albumin in tissue (K. Wang et al., 2019). The 3D vascularized proximal tubule (3D VasPT) was manufactured utilizing Pluronic ink deposited on modified ECM using gelatin and fibrin.

Bioinks to treat volumetric muscle wasting (VML) were produced from the tibialis anterior muscles and decellularized ECM (dECM) of the descending aortas of pigs (Cui et al., 2017). However, to closely mimic tissue formation, a branched vascular network capable of maintaining angiogenesis, remodeling, and function with the cell sources tried so far would be needed.

Bioprinting Techniques

Compared to conventional additive exhibitions utilizing cell-free platforms, bioprinting interests living cells during the precipitate method, which requires special protection due to their perceptiveness to temperature and mechanical stress, such as elevated pressure and shear tension and the pH biocompatibility of the surroundings. Accordingly, the 3D structure to be formed is foremost created operating CAD software to receive a 3D model. This design is then divided into layers, and each coating is disintegrated into a series of forms to fill the whole scaffolding.

There are four principal procedures in bioprinting: extrusion-based, drop-based, laser-based, and stereolithography bioprinting (Malda et al., 2013; Vijayavenkataraman et al., 2018). Each method has its necessities and components, which solve particular advantages and limitations. Furthermore, each technique assumes a different resolution range, imagination time, and strategy limitations (Moroni et al., 2018). In complement to the inherent specifications, bioprinting can act as the accompanying exhibition of one or more fabrics.

To manufacture vascular canals operating extrusion-based bioprinting (Bioplotting), most publications direct to cell-free inks deposited as a sacrificial hydrogel implanted in an ECM-like hydrogel to build a concave tubular scaffold after reduction (Kolesky et al., 2014; V. K. Lee et al., 2014). Then, virtually, the cells are crowded into a hand-released gel that envelopes the sacrificial ink. Here we think only of bioprinting, the technique that concerns the residue of a bioink and thus a cell-laden material, while others interconnected to cell-free material are regarded standard ink.

Extrusion Based Bioprinting

Bioplotting, the most standard technique, distributes a continuous filament from a cell-containing bioink employing a plunger, pneumatic system, or screw to create a layer-by-layer 3D structure. It is a technique that provides homogeneous cell distribution with the correct bioink deposition (resolution: >100 μm) and high processing speed. Moreover, due to the continuous deposition of bioinks, bioinks can achieve excellent structural integrity and very high cell density (Rider et al., 2018). However, it is essential to believe that more increased density bioinks guide to raised shear stress, reduced cell viability, and a limitation in smaller nozzle sizes. Furthermore, the pressure caused by the extrusion process can cause disruption or deterioration of cellular membranes, which affects cell viability; with excessive extrusion pressure, cell viability may decrease up to 40% (Bishop, 2017; Chang, 2008). Therefore, biomaterials should resemble natural ECM as much as possible to improve cell viability. Hydrogels must have a characteristic degree of immobility and biodegradability to allow cells to diffuse, limiting the selection of biomaterials (Kondiah, 2016; Mandrycky et al., 2015).

There are several techniques for extrusion bioprinting and each of them has its pros and cons. Pneumatic methods are often connected with delayed delivery due to squeezed gas, while they can sustain approvingly viscous biomaterials. Biomaterial extrusion offers better spatial control in screw-based systems, while piston-operated deposition provides better control overflow (Pati, 2015). A new strategy has emerged over the past decade to fabricate vascular structures. The templating technique, or altruistic templating, is a viable and pertinent method to fabricate tubular networks utilizing extrusion-based bioprinting. hMSCs were incorporated into the bioprinted matrix hydrogel, and HUVECs were perfused into the canal behind fibronectin injection to enable cell extension. Because a physiological tissue consists of several cell kinds performing in synergy, the ability to have a single tissue containing a vasculature that allows interchange between several embedded cell varieties makes this representative suitable for studying cell relations in a complicated domain.

Drop Based Bioprinting

A droplet is a motorized bioink for selective delivery of droplets passing through the piezoelectric or electrostatic pathway in electric or motorized droplets, piezoelectric or electric vehicle droplets, a departure from a substrate that has control over placement via a contactless system. Benefiting from advantages such as valve opening time, feed rate and delivery, droplet volume, and drop angle per drop support the average drop (Datta, 2017). This procedure supplies more decisiveness than bioprinting in extrusion (20–100 µm). In addition, the drip technique allows for the deposition of a live liquid in liquid or a low-viscosity hydrogel.

Strategies have been explored to construct structures using drop-forming bioprinting. For example, in three bioinks dispensed on three different printers: the first with 37°C HUVEC (10-12 million/ml by weight) 3% gelatin cross-solution (second with thrombin); and "Sesi contains 2.5% by weight fibrinogen with SMC (6 million/ml) (Schöneberg et al., 2018). This nest is impressive as they manage to reconstruct the three coatings of a blood vessel, regenerating tunica intima (endothelium), tunica environment (elastic SMCs) and tunica adventitia (fibroblast matrix). In addition, drop-based bioprinting is an effective process for creating tubular structures that mimic physiological arrangement, though underused in vascular bioprinting.

Laser-Assisted Bioprinting

Laser-Induced Forward Transfer (LIFT) or Laser-Assisted Bioprinting (LAB) utilizes a laser beating to isolate cells from a donor decline and position them on a specific substrate following a characteristic pattern (Moroni et al., 2018).

The donor slip or strip is often placed underneath the cell layer. It is a methal decline that is recognized as homogeneously as conceivable. After obtaining the laser pulsation from the lid of the donor decline, the metal immerses the power, inducing a bubble under the cell layer, leading to cell separation (Sasmal, 2018). This process integrates the most increased cell viability and heightened decisiveness (unique cell deposition) of the three previously mentioned strategies. Changing the density and consistency parameters of the bioink, the laser power, surface pressure, wettability, and air hole between the substrate and donor decreases make it likely to maintain the droplet importance accurately. However, this method is one of the smallest effective in volume per minute bioprinted and model practice (Moroni et al., 2018). Cell breaks should be packed below the donor slide and moist during the bioprinting procedure, demanding an incredibly elevated comparative humidity rate in the bioprinter compartment to control cell dehydration. LIFT's primary asset is the control and resolution of droplet buildup. This feature allows accumulating predirected cell lines to cause the development and maturing of cells following a typical pattern. Bioassembly is a biofabrication technique that produces a hierarchical structure via the automatic aggregation and rearrangement of material or cell, even called self-assembly. ECs can self-assemble and mature in a vascular-like grid in the existence of growth factors (Gruene, 2011). LAB can be employed as a prototype to direct the accumulation and growth of ECs, causing a self-assembly procedure leading to the construction of a pattern-specific vascular-like grid. LAB can also be operated to investigate cell-cell interchanges in collected surroundings.

Stereolithography Bioprinting

It is a selective additive production where a liquid photopolymer is cured by light-activated polymerization in a vessel. Stereolithography (SLA or SL), on the other hand, is a highly preferred vessel photopolymerization technique in biomedical applications, including surgical guides and dentistry, because it produces parts with high accuracy (Bajaj et al., 2013; Hunziker, 2002). Usually, features delivered by this method require reprocessing afterward. While delimited to photocrosslinkable polishes, advancements in the fabric retain developed the application of SLA technology to ceramic photopolymer composites (Pati et al., 2015). The application of vat polymerization for bioprinted vascular grafts should be attended by procedures that consider the subtraction of cytotoxic importance, such as uncured polish, from the function.

Conclusion

Stereolithography, laser-assisted, droplet-based, and extrusion-based multiple bioprinting techniques were used to obtain the in vitro vascular structure. While each is relatively successful, combined uses such as multi-material bioprinting are more attractive. In addition, thermal transitions, bioactivity/biocompatibility, or viscosity play an essential role in these modeling choices. In order to obtain a fully functional vascular network in the bioprinting of blood vessels, it has been created to make layers through different cell types and different proteins. The disadvantages of bioprinting are due to the pressure, material, cross-linking methods, or temperatures that must be used. Studies are based on the use of cells combined with a bioprinter mechanism that prevents cell death and is easier to manipulate, while challenging to translate into clinical scenarios.

Despite its advantages and disadvantages, it has been observed that the design and fabrication of tubular capillary networks and vessel reendothelialization and maturation are possible. However, the formation of vascular tissues and the construction of a multiscale vascular system have not been fully realized. More than one cell should be brought together spatially in a controlled manner. Still, it should be arranged to allow the formed tissue's differentiation, growth, and vasculogenesis. Most of the bioinks widely used today are chosen from natural bioinks, so it should be noted that it will offer many possibilities in synthetic inks.

References

Ahn, H., Ju, Y. M., Takahashi, H., Williams, D. F., Yoo, J. J., Lee, S. J., Okano, T., & Atala, A. (2015). Engineered small-diameter vascular grafts by combining cell sheet engineering and electrospinning technology. *Acta Biomaterialia*, *16*, 14–22. https://doi.org/10.1016/j.actbio.2015.01.030.

Bajaj, P., Marchwiany, D., Duarte, C., Bashir, R., Bajaj, P., Bashir, R., Marchwiany, D., & Duarte, C. (2013). Patterned three-dimensional encapsulation of embryonic stem cells using dielectrophoresis and stereolithography. *Advanced Healthcare Materials, 2,* 450–458. https://doi.org/10.1002/adhm.201200318.

Bishop E.S., M. S., P. M., L. H. H., L. M. J., W. J. M., A. G. A., H. T. C., R. R. R. (2017). 3-D bioprinting technologies in tissue engineering and regenerative medicine: Current and future trends. *Gene Funct. Dis.*, *4*, 185–195.

Bohorquez, M., Koch, C., Trygstad, T., & Pandit, N. (1999). A study of the temperature-dependent micellization of Pluronic F127. *Journal of Colloid and Interface Science*, *216*(1), 34–40. https://doi.org/10.1006/jcis.1999.6273.

Bose, S., Roy, M., & Bandyopadhyay, A. (2012). Recent advances in bone tissue engineering scaffolds. *Trends in Biotechnology*, *30*(10), 546–554. https://doi.org/10.1016/j.tibtech.2012.07.005.

Bourget, J.-M., Gauvin, R., Duchesneau, D., Remy, M., Auger, F. A., & Germain, L. (2015). Potential of newborn and adult stem cells for the production of vascular constructs using the living tissue sheet approach. *BioMed Research International*, *2015*, 168294. https://doi.org/10.1155/2015/168294.

Brandt, M. (2017). Laser additive manufacturing: materials, design, technologies, and applicati*ons*. In *Woodhead Publishing Series in Electronic and Optical Materials*. Woodhead Publishing. https://doi.org/10.1016/C2014-0-03891-9.

Bulanova, E. A., Koudan, E. V, Degosserie, J., Heymans, C., Pereira, F. D. A. S., Parfenov, V. A., Sun, Y., Wang, Q., Akhmedova, S. A., Sviridova, I. K., Sergeeva, N. S., Frank, G. A., Khesuani, Y. D., Pierreux, C. E., & Mironov, V. A. (2017). Bioprinting of a functional vascularized mouse thyroid gland construct. *Biofabrication*, *9*(3), 34105. https://doi.org/10.1088/1758-5090/aa7fdd.

Byambaa, B., Annabi, N., Yue, K., Trujillo-de Santiago, G., Alvarez, M. M., Jia, W., Kazemzadeh-Narbat, M., Shin, S. R., Tamayol, A., & Khademhosseini, A. (2017). Bioprinted osteogenic and vasculogenic patterns for engineering 3D bone tissue. *Advanced Healthcare Materials*, *6*(16). https://doi.org/10. 1002/adhm.201700015.

Carmeliet, P. (2000). Mechanisms of angiogenesis and arteriogenesis. *Nature Medicine*, *6*(4), 389–395. https://doi.org/10.1038/74651.

Carmeliet, P. (2004). Manipulating angiogenesis in medicine. *Journal of Internal Medicine*, *255*(5), 538–561. https://doi.org/10.1111/j.1365-2796.2003. 01297.x.

Carmeliet, P., & Jain, R. K. (2000). Angiogenesis in cancer and other diseases. *Nature*, *407*(6801), 249–257. https://doi.org/10.1038/35025220.

Catros, S., Guillemot, F., Nandakumar, A., Ziane, S., Moroni, L., Habibovic, P., van Blitterswijk, C., Rousseau, B., Chassande, O., Amédée, J., & Fricain, J.-C. (2012). Layer-by-layer tissue microfabrication supports cell proliferation in vitro and in vivo. *Tissue Engineering. Part C, Methods*, *18*(1), 62–70. https://doi.org/10.1089/ten.TEC.2011.0382.

Chang R., N. J., S. W. (2008). Effects of dispensing pressure and nozzle diameter on cell survival from solid freeform fabrication-based direct cell writing. *Tissue Eng*, *14*, 41–48.

Choi, Y.-J., Jun, Y.-J., Kim, D. Y., Yi, H.-G., Chae, S.-H., Kang, J., Lee, J., Gao, G., Kong, J.-S., Jang, J., Chung, W. K., Rhie, J.-W., & Cho, D.-W. (2019). A 3D cell printed muscle construct with tissue-derived bioink for the treatment of volumetric muscle loss. *Biomaterials*, *206*, 160–169. https://doi.org/10.1016/j.biomaterials. 2019.03.036.

Clark, J. M., & Glagov, S. (1985). Transmural organization of the arterial media. The lamellar unit revisited. *Arteriosclerosis*, *5*(1), 19–34. https://doi.org/10.1161/01.atv. 5.1.19.

Cross, M. J., & Claesson-Welsh, L. (2001). FGF and VEGF function in angiogenesis: signalling pathways, biological responses, and therapeutic inhibition. *Trends in Pharmacological Sciences*, *22*(4), 201–207. https://doi.org/https://doi.org/10.1016/ S0165-6147(00)01676-X.

Cui, H., Nowicki, M., Fisher, J. P., & Zhang, L. G. (2017). 3D bioprinting for organ regeneration. *Advanced Healthcare Materials*, *6*(1), 1–29. https://doi.org/10.1002/ adhm.201601118.

Cui, H., Zhu, W., Nowicki, M., Zhou, X., Khademhosseini, A., & Zhang, L. G. (2016). Hierarchical Fabrication of Engineered Vascularized Bone Biphasic Constructs via Dual 3D Bioprinting: Integrating Regional Bioactive Factors into Architectural Design. *Advanced Healthcare Materials*, *5*(17), 2174–2181. https://doi.org/10.1002/ adhm.201600505.

Datta P., A. B., O. I. T. (2017). Bioprinting for vascular and vascularized tissue biofabrication. *Acta Biomater*, *51*, 1–20.

Diban, N., Haimi, S., Bolhuis-Versteeg, L., Teixeira, S., Miettinen, S., Poot, A., Grijpma, D., & Stamatialis, D. (2013). Hollow fibers of poly(lactide-co-glycolide) and poly(ε-caprolactone) blends for vascular tissue engineering applications. *Acta Biomaterialia*, *9*(5), 6450–6458. https://doi.org/10.1016/j. actbio.2013.01.005.

Druecke, D., Langer, S., Lamme, E., Pieper, J., Ugarkovic, M., Steinau, H. U., & Homann, H. H. (2004). Neovascularization of poly(ether ester) block copolymer scaffolds in vivo: long-term investigations using intravital fluorescent microscopy. *Journal of Biomedical Materials Research. Part A*, *68*(1), 10–18. https://doi.org/10.1002/jbm.a. 20016.

Feng, F., & Ye, L. (2011). Morphologies and mechanical properties of polylactide/ thermoplastic polyurethane elastomer blends. *Journal of Applied Polymer Science*, *119*(5), 2778–2783. https://doi.org/10.1002/app.32863.

Freiman, A., Shandalov, Y., Rozenfeld, D., Shor, E., Segal, S., Ben-David, D., Meretzki, S., Egozi, D., & Levenberg, S. (2016). Adipose-derived endothelial and mesenchymal stem cells enhance vascular network formation on three-dimensional constructs in vitro. *Stem Cell Research & Therapy*, *7*, 5. https://doi.org/10.1186/ s13287-015-0251-6.

Frid, M. G., Kale, V. A., & Stenmark, K. R. (2002). Mature vascular endothelium can give rise to smooth muscle cells via endothelial-mesenchymal transdifferentiation: in vitro analysis. *Circulation Research*, *90*(11), 1189–1196. https://doi.org/10.1161/01.res.00 00021432.70309.28.

Gao, G., Park, J. Y., Kim, B. S., Jang, J., & Cho, D.-W. (2018). Coaxial Cell Printing of Freestanding, Perfusable, and Functional In Vitro Vascular Models for Recapitulation of Native Vascular Endothelium Pathophysiology. *Advanced Healthcare Materials*, *7*(23), e1801102. https://doi.org/10.1002/ adhm.201801102.

Gomes, S., Leonor, I. B., Mano, J. F., Reis, R. L., & Kaplan, D. L. (2012). Natural and genetically engineered proteins for tissue engineering. *Progress in Polymer Science*, *37*(1), 1–17. https://doi.org/https://doi.org/10.1016/j. progpolymsci.2011.07.003.

Gruene M., P. M., H. C., D. S., S. S., D. A., K. L., W. M., J. S., H. A., et al. (2011). Laser Printing of three-dimensional multicellular arrays for studies of cell-cell and cell–environment interactions. *Tissue Eng. Part C: Methods.*, *17*, 973–982.

Gungor-Ozkerim, P. S., Inci, I., Zhang, Y. S., Khademhosseini, A., & Dokmeci, M. R. (2018). Bioinks for 3D bioprinting: an overview. *Biomaterials Science*, *6*(5), 915–946. https://doi.org/10.1039/c7bm00765e.

Hoch, E., Tovar, G. E. M., & Borchers, K. (2014). Bioprinting of artificial blood vessels: current approaches towards a demanding goal. *European Journal of Cardio-Thoracic Surgery*, *46*(5), 767–778. https://doi.org/10.1093/ejcts/ ezu242.

Hunziker, E. B. (2002). Articular cartilage repair: basic science and clinical progress. A review of the current status and prospects. *Osteoarthritis and Cartilage*, *10*(6), 432–463. https://doi.org/10.1053/JOCA.2002.0801.

Jungst, T., Smolan, W., Schacht, K., Scheibel, T., & Groll, J. (2016). Strategies and molecular design criteria for 3d printable hydrogels. *Chemical Reviews*, *116*(3), 1496–1539. https://doi.org/10.1021/acs.chemrev.5b00303.

Kolesky, D. B., Truby, R. L., Sydney Gladman, A., Busbee, T. A., Homan, K. A., Lewis, J. A., Kolesky, D. B., Truby, R. L., Gladman, A. S., Busbee, T., Homan, K. A., & Lewis, J. A. (2014). 3D bioprinting of vascularized, heterogeneous cell-laden tissue constructs. *Advanced Materials, 26*(9), 3124–3130. https://doi.org/10.1002/adma.20 1305506.

Kondiah P.J., C. Y. E., K. P. P. D., M. T., K. P., du T. L. C., P. v. (2016). A review of injectable polymeric hydrogel systems for application in bone tissue engineering. *Molecules*, *21*, 1–31.

Kreimendahl, F., Köpf, M., Thiebes, A. L., Duarte Campos, D. F., Blaeser, A., Schmitz-Rode, T., Apel, C., Jockenhoevel, S., & Fischer, H. (2017). Three-dimensional printing and angiogenesis: tailored agarose-type i collagen blends comprise three-dimensional printability and angiogenesis potential for tissue-engineered substitutes. *Tissue Engineering Part C: Methods*, *23*(10), 604–615. https://doi.org/10.1089/ten. tec.2017.0234.

Krogh, A. (1922). *The Anatomy and Physiology of Capillaries*. Yale University Press.

Lee, J. W., Choi, Y.-J., Yong, W.-J., Pati, F., Shim, J.-H., Kang, K. S., Kang, I.-H., Park, J., & Cho, D.-W. (2016). Development of a 3D cell printed construct considering angiogenesis for liver tissue engineering. *Biofabrication*, *8*(1), 15007. https://doi.org /10.1088/1758-5090/8/1/015007.

Lee, V. K., Kim, D. Y., Ngo, H., Lee, Y., Seo, L., Yoo, S.-S., Vincent, P. A., & Dai, G. (2014). Creating perfused functional vascular channels using 3D bio-printing technology. *Biomaterials*, *35*(28), 8092–8102. https://doi.org/10.1016/j.biomaterials. 2014.05.083.

Lin, R.-Z., & Chang, H.-Y. (2008). Recent advances in three-dimensional multicellular spheroid culture for biomedical research. *Biotechnology Journal*, *3*(9–10), 1172–1184. https://doi.org/10.1002/biot.200700228.

Lovett, M., Lee, K., Edwards, A., & Kaplan, D. L. (2009). Vascularization strategies for tissue engineering. *Tissue Engineering. Part B, Reviews*, *15*(3), 353–370. https://doi. org/10.1089/ten.TEB.2009.0085.

Maguire, E. M., Xiao, Q., & Xu, Q. (2017). Differentiation and application of induced pluripotent stem cell-derived vascular smooth muscle cells. *Arteriosclerosis, Thrombosis, and Vascular Biology, 37*(11), 2026–2037. https://doi.org/10.1161/ATVBAHA.117.309196.

Malda, J., Rouwkema, J., Martens, D. E., Le Comte, E. P., Kooy, F. K., Tramper, J., van Blitterswijk, C. A., & Riesle, J. (2004). Oxygen gradients in tissue-engineered PEGT/PBT cartilaginous constructs: measurement and modeling. *Biotechnology and Bioengineering, 86*(1), 9–18. https://doi.org/10.1002/bit. 20038.

Malda, J., Visser, J., Melchels, F. P., Jüngst, T., Hennink, W. E., A Dhert, W. J., Groll, J., Hutmacher, D. W., Malda, J., Visser, J., Melchels, F. P., A Dhert, W. J., & Hutmacher, D. W. (2013). 25th anniversary article: engineering hydrogels for biofabrication. *Adv. Mater, 25*, 5011–5028. https://doi.org/10.1002/adma. 201302042.

Mandrycky, C., Wang, Z., Kim, K., & Kim, D.-H. (2015). 3D bioprinting for engineering complex tissues. *Biotechnol Adv.*, 34(4):422-434. https://doi.org/10.1016/j.biotechadv.2015.12.011.

Marc, T. (1922). Anatomy and physiology of the circulatory and ventilatory systems. In *Biomathematical and Biomechanical Modeling of the Circulatory and Ventilatory, 6.* Systems. Springer Publications.

McAnulty, R. J. (2007). Fibroblasts and myofibroblasts: their source, function, and role in disease. *The International Journal of Biochemistry & Cell Biology, 39*(4), 666–671. https://doi.org/10.1016/j.biocel.2006.11.005.

Melchels, F. P. W., Domingos, M. A. N., Klein, T. J., Malda, J., Bartolo, P. J., & Hutmacher, D. W. (2012). Additive manufacturing of tissues and organs. *Progress in Polymer Science, 37*(8), 1079–1104. https://doi.org/https://doi.org/10.1016/j.progpolymsci.2011.11.007.

Mercado-Pagán, Á. E., Kang, Y., Findlay, M. W., & Yang, Y. (2015). Development and evaluation of elastomeric hollow fiber membranes as small-diameter vascular graft substitutes. *Materials Science & Engineering. C, Materials for Biological Applications, 49*, 541–548. https://doi.org/10.1016/j. msec.2015.01.051.

Miller, J. S., Stevens, K. R., Yang, M. T., Baker, B. M., Nguyen, D.-H. T., Cohen, D. M., Toro, E., Chen, A. A., Galie, P. A., Yu, X., Chaturvedi, R., Bhatia, S. N., & Chen, C. S. (2012). Rapid casting of patterned vascular networks for perfusable engineered three-dimensional tissues. *Nature Materials, 11*(9), 768–774. https://doi.org/10.1038/nmat3357.

Mirea, O., Donoiu, I., & Pleşea, I. E. (2012). Arterial aging: A brief review. *Romanian Journal of Morphology and Embryology, 53*(3), 473–477.

Moroni, L., Boland, T., Burdick, J. A., de Maria, C., Derby, B., Forgacs, G., Groll, J., Li, Q., Malda, J., Mironov, V. A., Mota, C., Nakamura, M., Shu, W., Takeuchi, S., Woodfield, T. B. F., Xu, T., Yoo, J. J., & Vozzi, G. (2018). Biofabrication: a guide to technology and terminology. *Trends in Biotechnology, 36*(4), 384–402. https://doi.org/10.1016/J.TIBTECH.2017. 10.015.

Norotte, C., Marga, F. S., Niklason, L. E., & Forgacs, G. (2009). Scaffold-free vascular tissue engineering using bioprinting. *Biomaterials, 30*(30), 5910–5917. https://doi.org/https://doi.org/10.1016/j.biomaterials.2009.06.034.

Novosel, E. C., Kleinhans, C., & Kluger, P. J. (2011). Vascularization is the key challenge in tissue engineering. *Advanced Drug Delivery Reviews*, *63*(4–5), 300–311. https://doi.org/10.1016/j.addr.2011.03.004.

Organdonor.gov. (n.d.). *U.S. Department of Health and Social Services*. Retrieved October 28, 2016, from http://www.organdonor.gov/statistics-stories statistics.html.

Paschalaki, K. E., & Randi, A. M. (2018). Recent advances in endothelial colony forming cells toward their use in clinical translation. *Frontiers in Medicine*, *5*, 295. https://doi.org/10.3389/fmed.2018.00295.

Pati F., J. J., L. J. W., C. D. W. (2015). Extrusion bioprinting. In Y. J. J. Atala A. (Ed.), In *Essentials of 3D Biofabrication and Translation.* (pp. 123–152). Academic Press.

Pati, F., Jang, J., Lee, J. W., & Cho, D. W. (2015). Extrusion Bioprinting. *Essentials of 3D Biofabrication and Translation*, 123–152. https://doi.org/10.1016/B978-0-12-80097 2-7.00007-4.

Paulsen, S. J., & Miller, J. S. (2015). Tissue vascularization through 3D printing: Will technology bring us flow? *Developmental Dynamics : An Official Publication of the American Association of Anatomists*, *244*(5), 629–640. https://doi.org/10.1002/dvd y.24254.

Pirlo, R. K., Wu, P., Liu, J., & Ringeisen, B. (2012). PLGA/hydrogel biopapers as a stackable substrate for printing HUVEC networks via BioLP. *Biotechnology and Bioengineering*, *109*(1), 262–273. https://doi.org/10.1002/ bit.23295.

Prince, E. A., & Ahn, S. H. (2013). Basic vascular neuroanatomy of the brain and spine: what the general interventional radiologist needs to know. *Semin Intervent Radiol*, *30*(03), 234–239.

Qiu, Y., Zhang, N., Kang, Q., An, Y., & Wen, X. (2009). Fabrication of permeable tubular constructs from chemically modified chitosan with enhanced antithrombogenic property. *Journal of Biomedical Materials Research Part B: Applied Biomaterials*, *90B*(2), 668–678. https://doi.org/https://doi.org/10. 1002/jbm.b.31333.

Rider P., Kačarević Ž. P., Alkildani S., Retnasingh S., & Barbeck M. (2018). Bioprinting of tissue engineering scaffolds. *J. Tissue Eng*, *9*, 1–16. https://doi.org/10.1177/2041 731418802090.

Rosa, S., Praça, C., Pitrez, P. R., Gouveia, P. J., Aranguren, X. L., Ricotti, L., & Ferreira, L. S. (2019). Functional characterization of iPSC-derived arterial- and venous-like endothelial cells. *Scientific Reports*, *9*(1), 3826. https://doi.org/10.1038/s41598-019-40417-9.

Rouwkema, J., & Khademhosseini, A. (2016). Vascularization and angiogenesis in tissue engineering: beyond creating static networks. *Trends in Biotechnology*, *34*(9), 733–745. https://doi.org/10.1016/j.tibtech.2016.03.002.

Santos, M. I., & Reis, R. L. (2010). Vascularization in bone tissue engineering: physiology, current strategies, major hurdles, and future challenges. *Macromolecular Bioscience*, *10*(1), 12–27. https://doi.org/10.1002/mabi. 200900107.

Santos, M. I., Tuzlakoglu, K., Fuchs, S., Gomes, M. E., Peters, K., Unger, R. E., Piskin, E., Reis, R. L., & Kirkpatrick, C. J. (2008). Endothelial cell colonization and angiogenic potential of combined nano- and micro-fibrous scaffolds for bone tissue engineering. *Biomaterials*, *29*(32), 4306–4313. https://doi.org/10.1016/j.biomaterials.2008.07.033.

Sasmal P., D. P., W. Y., O. I. T. (2018). 3D bioprinting for modelling vasculature. *Microphysiol. Syst.*, *2*(9), 1–17.

Schöneberg, J., de Lorenzi, F., Theek, B., Blaeser, A., Rommel, D., Kuehne, A. J. C., Kießling, F., & Fischer, H. (2018). Engineering biofunctional in vitro vessel models using a multilayer bioprinting technique. *Scientific Reports*, *8*(1), 10430. https://doi.org/10.1038/s41598-018-28715-0.

Sekine, H., Shimizu, T., Yang, J., Kobayashi, E., & Okano, T. (2006). Pulsatile myocardial tubes fabricated with cell sheet engineering. *Circulation*, *114*(1_supplement), I-87-I–93. https://doi.org/10.1161/CIRCULATIONAHA. 105.000273.

Skardal, A., Zhang, J., McCoard, L., Oottamasathien, S., & Prestwich, G. D. (2010a). Dynamically Crosslinked Gold Nanoparticle – Hyaluronan Hydrogels. *Advanced Materials*, *22*(42), 4736–4740. https://doi.org/https://doi.org/10.1002/adma.201001436.

Skardal, A., Zhang, J., McCoard, L., Xu, X., Oottamasathien, S., & Prestwich, G. D. (2010b). Photocrosslinkable hyaluronan-gelatin hydrogels for two-step bioprinting. *Tissue Engineering Part A*, *16*(8), 2675–2685. https://doi.org/10.1089/ten.tea.2009.0798.

Skardal, A., Zhang, J., & Prestwich, G. D. (2010c). Bioprinting vessel-like constructs using hyaluronan hydrogels crosslinked with tetrahedral polyethylene glycol tetracrylates. *Biomaterials*, *31*(24), 6173–6181. https://doi.org/https://doi.org/10.1016/j.biomaterials.2010.04.045.

Stahl, P. J., Chan, T. R., Shen, Y.-I., Sun, G., Gerecht, S., & Yu, S. M. (2014). Capillary network-like organization of endothelial cells in pegda scaffolds encoded with angiogenic signals via triple helical hybridization. *Advanced Functional Materials*, *24*(21), 3213–3225. https://doi.org/https://doi.org/10.1002/adfm. 201303217.

Tijore, A., Behr, J.-M., Irvine, S. A., Baisane, V., & Venkatraman, S. (2018). Bioprinted gelatin hydrogel platform promotes smooth muscle cell contractile phenotype maintenance. *Biomedical Microdevices*, *20*(2), 32. https://doi.org/10.1007/s10544-018-0274-8.

Tremblay, P.-L., Hudon, V., Berthod, F., Germain, L., & Auger, F. A. (2005). Inosculation of tissue-engineered capillaries with the host's vasculature in a reconstructed skin transplanted on mice. *American Journal of Transplantation : Official Journal of the American Society of Transplantation and the American Society of Transplant Surgeons*, *5*(5), 1002–1010. https://doi.org/10.1111/j.1600-6143.2005.00790.x.

Veith, F. J., Moss, C. M., Sprayregen, S., & Montefusco, C. (1979). Preoperative saphenous venography in arterial reconstructive surgery of the lower extremity. *Surgery*, *85*(3), 253–256.

Vijayavenkataraman, S., Yan, W.-C., Lu, W. F., Wang, C.-H., Hsi Fuh, J. Y., & Hsi Fuh. (2018). 3D bioprinting of tissues and organs for regenerative medicine. *Advanced Drug Delivery Reviews*, *132*, 296–332.

Visconti, R. P., Kasyanov, V., Gentile, C., Zhang, J., Markwald, R. R., & Mironov, V. (2010). Towards organ printing: engineering an intra-organ branched vascular tree. *Expert Opinion on Biological Therapy*, *10*(3), 409–420. https://doi.org/10.1517/14712590903563352.

Wang, G., Jacquet, L., Karamariti, E., & Xu, Q. (2015). Origin and differentiation of vascular smooth muscle cells. *The Journal of Physiology*, *593*(14), 3013–3030. https://doi.org/10.1113/JP270033.

Wang, K., Lin, R.-Z., & Melero-Martin, J. M. (2019). Bioengineering human vascular networks: trends and directions in endothelial and perivascular cell sources. *Cellular and Molecular Life Sciences : CMLS*, *76*(3), 421–439. https://doi.org/10.1007/s00018-018-2939-0.

Wang, W., Hu, J., He, C., Nie, W., Feng, W., Qiu, K., Zhou, X., Gao, Y., & Wang, G. (2015). Heparinized PLLA/PLCL nanofibrous scaffold for potential engineering of small-diameter blood vessel: tunable elasticity and anticoagulation property. *Journal of Biomedical Materials Research. Part A*, *103*(5), 1784–1797. https://doi.org/10.1002/jbm.a.35315.

Wu, P. K., & Ringeisen, B. R. (2010). Development of human umbilical vein endothelial cell ({HUVEC}) and human umbilical vein smooth muscle cell ({HUVSMC}) branch/stem structures on hydrogel layers via biological laser printing ({BioLP}). *Biofabrication*, *2*(1), 14111. https://doi.org/10.1088/1758-5082/2/1/014111.

Yang, S., Leong, K.-F., Du, Z., & Chua, C.-K. (2002). The design of scaffolds for use in tissue engineering. Part II. Rapid prototyping techniques. *Tissue Engineering*, *8*(1), 1–11. https://doi.org/10.1089/107632702753503009.

Zhang, W., Wray, L. S., Rnjak-Kovacina, J., Xu, L., Zou, D., Wang, S., Zhang, M., Dong, J., Li, G., Kaplan, D. L., & Jiang, X. (2015). Vascularization of hollow channel-modified porous silk scaffolds with endothelial cells for tissue regeneration. *Biomaterials*, *56*, 68–77. https://doi.org/10.1016/j.biomaterials. 2015.03.053.

Zhao, H., Chen, Y., Shao, L., Xie, M., Nie, J., Qiu, J., Zhao, P., Ramezani, H., Fu, J., Ouyang, H., & He, Y. (2018). Airflow-assisted 3D bioprinting of human heterogeneous microspheroidal organoids with microfluidic nozzle. *Small (Weinheim an Der Bergstrasse, Germany)*, *14*(39), e1802630. https://doi.org/10.1002/ smll.201802630.

Chapter 8

Bioprinting for Tissue Engineering

Ömer Bozduman[1,*], MD
and Ömer Cahit Çıtır[2], MD
[1]Department of Orthopedics and Traumatology,
University of Samsun, Samsun, Turkey
[2]Department of Orthopedics and Traumatology,
University of Tokat Gaziosmanpaşa, Tokat, Turkey

Abstract

3D printers are used in many fields from engineering to health today. Along with the incredible progress in 3D printing technology, it has also provided new opportunities for healthcare providers. One of them is 3D bone tissue engineering.

There are many surgeries that are produced with 3D technology and placed in the body, such as the replacement of large bone defects. The most common of these are bony areas that occupy a large volume such as long bone or pelvis, which are removed in malignant tumor surgery, closure of bone defects formed after operations such as trauma tumor surgery in the skull, or creation of the mandible in jaw surgery (McCulloch et al., 2021; Shen et al., 2020; Dupret-Bories et al., 2018).

A subject where 3D bone engineering is frequently used is understanding preoperative deformity by surgeons and creating reality simulations. The creation of images obtained with 3D CTs taken before spinal deformity surgery or malignant tumor surgeries, where a large bone tissue loss is expected, with 3D printers and surgical planning accordingly, are widely used today.

---

* Corresponding Author's Email: omerbozduman@gmail.com.

In: Bioprinting the Human
Editors: Soner Şahin and Kenan Demir
ISBN: 978-1-68507-993-2

In this study, we will provide information on the place of 3D bone engineering, the difficulties encountered in its development stage and still ongoing, and the estimated usage areas of this technology in our lives in the future.

Keywords: 3D bioprinting, bone tissue engineering, scaffold

Introduction

Scaffolds are the foundation of bone tissue engineering. It is essential to use appropriate biochemical and physicochemical biomaterials in the creation of scaffolds. The tissues produced with this technology are used to replace or improve bone and surrounding tissue. In this respect, progress is inevitable in the fields of interest in orthopedics. The tissue obtained with this technology can be used as a graft for the repair of a patient's bone. The underlying scaffold structure is structurally similar to bone. This structure conforms to the required composition and porosity. When the scaffold structure is created, existing bone tissue or stem cells can be used. These two methods have proven to be successful (Fielding G et al., 2013; De Mori et al., 2018).

The main purpose of using this technology in bone tissue engineering is to repair the bone defect formed for any reason by tissue engineering. In the treatment of bone defects with traditional methods, structural or functional changes develop in bone tissue. In bone tissue engineering, the aim is to repair the bone defect by producing an artificial bone structure with the appropriate shape, size, mechanical strength, and properties. In this sense, it is superior to traditional techniques (Chen G., 2015; Hamlet et al., 2017).

3D printing technology was developed primarily for industrial use. Later, it was used in the medical field. With the realization that 3D printing technology can be used in tissue damage or organ defects that may develop due to various reasons such as infection, trauma, and congenital anomalies during human life, it has paved the way for many developments. Bone tissue engineering based on this technology is a multidisciplinary approach that uses a combination of cells and biomaterials to restore the required tissue function.

The first step in obtaining bone tissue with 3D printing is to obtain data of the defected bone area with CT or magnetic resonance imaging. The scaffold design is completed by shaping the obtained data in an electronic environment with appropriate software programs. In this way, a scaffold that is fully compatible with the shape, size, mechanically, and biologically is produced for the required area. The next step in the scaffold structure, which is produced after the selection of the appropriate material, is the placement of cells and tissues on the scaffold. The finalized scaffold is surgically implanted into the patient.

Creating 3D Bone

Trauma, excision of malignancy, etc. of bone tissue that has the ability to regenerate. In some cases, a defect may develop in sizes that exceed its capacity. The first method that comes to mind for the repair of bone defects is autologous tissue transplants. However, it is known to have complications such as the need for secondary surgery in the donor area, infection, deformity, scar tissue, and chronic pain (Qasim et al., 2019; Javaid and Haleem, 2019a; Haleem and Javaid, 2019). In addition, grafts of limited shape and size can be obtained.

Another technique used in the repair of bone defects is the use of allografts. Graft tissue is usually obtained from cadavers. Like autografts, allografts are tissue compatible. Cortical, cancellous, and combined grafts can be obtained. However, unlike autograft, there is a risk of immune reaction in this technique. There is also a risk of infection after surgery. Since it undergoes processes such as freezing and irradiation before application, its osteo-inductive properties are also less than those of autografts (Javaid and Haleem, 2019b; Amini et al., 2012; Fielding et al., 2013).

In addition to the methods mentioned, there are techniques such as distraction osteogenesis, bone morphogenic proteins (BMP), and filling of defects with cement. Although they are used in clinical practice, none of these techniques alone has all the features required for a perfect graft.

The ideal graft tissue to be used in the repair of bone defects; It should be highly osteoinductive, have angiogenic potential, be biologically safe, have no shape and size restrictions, be accessible when needed, cost-effective, and not cause additional morbidity to the patient. It has been shown that 3D printing technology can be a new treatment method that includes all these features. It is a promising method for bone defect repair using bone tissue engineering, since regeneration will proceed with the patient's own bone tissue and there are no risks of secondary surgical intervention.

One of the surgeries in which 3D bone printing technology is frequently used is malignant pelvic bone loss, where large bone defects can occur (Figure 1).

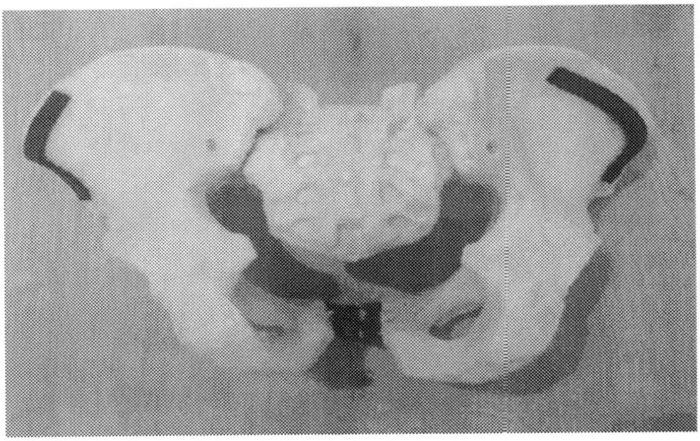

Figure 1. Pelvis image produced with 3D printing technology.

Scaffolds are the basis for bone tissue engineering. A 3-dimensional structure is obtained that allows cells to attach to bone tissue through scaffolds (Vaishya et al., 2018). The quality of the scaffold is decided on based on the important properties of these structures, such as the number of pores, the pore volume, the pore size, the chemical properties and the mechanical strength. To obtain a new and functional bone tissue, the structure and mechanics of bone tissue must be well understood.

Various methods are available to construct porous bone scaffolds, which are the structural basis of bone tissue engineering. Solvent casting, foaming gel, chemical foaming, and freeze drying are the main methods (Bose et al., 2017; Witte et al., 2018). Different types of 3D printing technologies are used depending on the region to be printed and the material desired to be used. Similarly, depending on the part planned to be produced, materials such as plastic, gypsum powder, ceramic, metal, sand, aluminide, polyether ether ketone (PEEK) and graphene are used (de Azevedo Gonçalves Mota et al., 2016; Sa et al., 2018).

Tissue regeneration is increased by producing biological tissues and organs with 3D printing. Inkjet 3D printers lead to hudge innovation in bone tissue engineering. With this technology, proper distribution of cells on the 3D Scaffold is facilitated. Bioinks can be used in cases where effective tissue regeneration or reconstruction is required (Seitz et al., 2005; Haleem and Javaid, 2018).

The bone structure consists of 2 different layers: spongy and cortical. The inner layer has a spongy part and the outer layer has a hard cortical part. Both layers have self-healing capacity. However, with this new technology, it is intended to facilitate the treatment of bone-related diseases. During bone tissue formation, very important benefits of 3D printing technology are seen in the stages of adhesion, proliferation, differentiation, and cell migration (Seitz et al., 2005; Haleem and Javaid, 2018).

The first step in obtaining bone tissue with 3D printing is to obtain data of the defected bone area with CT or magnetic resonance imaging. The scaffold design is completed by shaping the obtained data in an electronic environment with appropriate software programs. In this way, a scaffold that is fully compatible with the shape, size, mechanically, and biologically is produced for the required area. The next step in the scaffold structure, which is produced after the selection of the appropriate material, is the placement of cells and tissues on the scaffold. The finalized scaffold is surgically implanted into the patient.

Bıomaterıals

There are 3 basic structures that are taken as a basis when obtaining artificial bone. The first of these is the bone scaffold. It forms a bone-like structure in terms of physical and mechanical stability. This structure allows for cell attachment and migration. It mediates the retention of biochemicals and other essential substances. The scaffold structure helps the cell integrate into bone tissue and fulfills the needs of bone tissue (Gao et al., 2014).

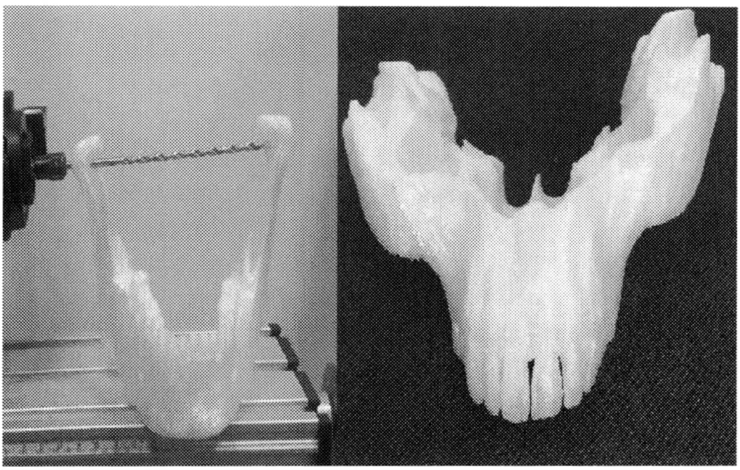

Figure 2. Mandible and maxilla images produced with 3D printing technology.

Another basic structure is the cell. The cell is the basis of life and is tissue-specific. Cells support tissue and maintain specialized functions. With 3D printing, it is aimed at supporting cells and thus maintaining function (Duarte Campos et al., 2016; Cidonio et al., 2019).

The final building block of bone tissue engineering is growth factors. There are different growth factors, such as fibroblast growth factor (FGF), vascular endothelial growth factor (VEGF), and bone morphogenic proteins (BMP).

Another of the most important stages of bone tissue engineering is the selection of suitable biomaterials for scaffold production. It is important that the selected biomaterial is mechanically strong enough for the scaffold produced to be surgically implanted and to function in the bone tissue.

To support the growth of cells and tissues on the scaffold, the biomaterial to be selected must be chemically suitable. Bioceramics, polymers, and hybrid materials are examples of these materials and are directly related to positive clinical outcomes.

Osteoinductive Materials

They are called smart biomaterials. They induce ectopic bone formation by stimulating surrounding tissue (Blokhuis and Arts, 2011; Barradas et al., 2011; Habibovic and de Groot, 2007). Although the high potential of these materials is known, how they function biologically has not been fully elucidated. Examples of these materials are synthetic and natural ceramics (hydroxyapatite (HA)), various calcium phosphate compositions, and their combinations (i.e., HA/poly(lactic-coglycolic acid) (PLGA).

The chemical properties of biomaterials play an important role in osteoinduction, as well as in the porosity and surface topography of the implant. It is not yet known exactly which of these two important factors contributes more to osteoinduction (Barradas et al., 2011).

Hybrid Materials: Ceramics and many various natural and synthetic polymers are biomaterials used in bone tissue engineering. The fact that not all of the physical, chemical, and biological properties required for bone tissue scaffolding cannot be found in a single biomaterial has led to the development of hybrid materials. As a result, copolymers, polymer-polymer mixtures, and polymer-ceramic combinations have been developed (Saad et al., 2000; Nukavarapu et al., 2009; Wahl and Czernuszka, 2006).

Hydrogels: Because of their physical properties, they have long been used in tissue engineering. They are materials with very high biocompatibility. They successfully mimic the structure of the extracellular matrix. They support tissue regeneration by providing various bioactive substances. Naturally sourced collagen and gelatins, synthetic poly(ethylene glycol) materials, and poly(vinyl alcohol) based hydrogels are used in bone tissue engineering (Slaughter et al., 2009; Park, 2011).

Immunmodulator Biomaterials: It is aimed to provide high bone repair and regeneration with these materials, which function by modulating and manipulating the immune system. It is based on the strategy of modifying the host's immune response to the requirements of bone tissue regeneration, rather than suppressing it. Modulation of the surface of the biomaterial, artificial extracellular matrix, and incorporation of bioactive molecules are examples of these strategies. Corticosteroids, cytokine-specific agents, prostaglandins, non-steroidal anti-inflammatory drugs, prostaglandin analogs, and growth hormones are areas of interest in immunobioengineering (Kou and Babensee, 2011; Anderson et al., 2008; Sheller et al., 2004).

Another important parameter in the selection of biomaterials is the biological structure. It should biologically support cell growth and form a new matrix and should not cause toxicity. In this way, complete and perfect bone tissue regeneration is achieved. Another requirement for the suitability of the biological structure is that it is biodegradable. The scaffold structure produced by 3D printing is not a permanent implant. It should stimulate the cells in it to perform their routine functions, and it should be biodegradable at the appropriate time, enabling the cells to grow and produce their own extracellular matrix. To meet the needs of the cells it hosts, the scaffold must be in a structure that supports vascular growth.

Conclusion

With recent developments, the integration of miRNA therapy into the 3D printing field is on the agenda. miRNAs are small noncoding RNAs. They regulate post-transcriptional gene expression. In mouse experiments applied this way, osteogenic induction was observed to increase and bone defects closed (Haleem and Javaid, 2019c; Moncal et al., 2019; Tanataweethum, 2015).

As one of the current developments, it is tried to use the scaffold structure, which contains many pores, by filling it with collagen. Compared to conventional scaffold structures, it has been observed that many more cells can be loaded on the scaffold. As a result, an increase in tissue regeneration and extracellular matrix production has been reported (Haleem and Javaid, 2019c; Moncal et al., 2019; Tanataweethum, 2015).

When the clinical use areas are examined, the repair of bone defects comes first. New tissues created by 3D printing allow bone defects to be removed. Due to the specific shape, size, and function of bone tissue produced according to needs, complex surgical processes can be avoided.

Tissue and organ damage develops for various reasons throughout human life. Tissue engineering has provided great innovations in order to repair damaged tissues and organs or to obtain new ones. The structures produced with 3D printing are used for preoperative planning, diagnosis, and education, as well as for treatment. Bone tissue engineering also serves all these purposes. Regeneration of bone defects is a very challenging process with conventional techniques. However, it seems possible to obtain lower-risk and more satisfactory results with bone tissue engineering.

References

Amini, A. R., Laurencin, C. T., Nukavarapu, S. P. (2012). Bone tissue engineering: recent advances and challenges. *Crit. Rev. Biomed. Eng.*, 40(5), 363-408.

Anderson, J., Rodriguez, A., Chang, D. (2008). Foreign body reaction to biomaterials. *Semin. Immunol.*, 20(2), 86-100.

Barradas, A. M., Yuan, H., van Blitterswijk, C. A., Habibo-vic, P. (2011). Osteoinductive biomaterials: Current knowledge of properties, experimental models, and biological mechanisms. *Eur. Cell Mater.*, 21, 407-429.

Blokhuis, T. J., Arts, J. J. (2011). Bioactive and osteoinductive bone graft substitutes: definitions, facts and myths. *Injury*, 42(2), S26-S29.

Bose, S., Tarafder, S., Bandyopadhyay, A. (2017). Effect of chemistry on osteogenesis and angiogenesis towards bone tissue engineering using 3D printed scaffolds. *Ann. Biomed. Eng.*, 45(1), 261-272.

Chen, G. (2015). 3D scaffolds with different stiffness but the same microstructure for bone tissue engineering. *ACS Appl. Mater. Interfaces*, 7(29), 15790-15802.

Cidonio, G., Glinka, M., Dawson, J. I., Oreffo, R. O. C. (2019). The cell in the ink: Improving biofabrication by printing stem cells for skeletal regenerative medicine. *Biomaterials*, 209, 10-24.

de Azevedo Gonçalves Mota, R. C., da Silva, E. O., de Lima, F. F., de Menezes, L. R. and Thiele, A. C. S. (2016) 3D Printed scaffolds as a new perspective for bone tissue regeneration: literature review. *Materials Sciences and Applications*, 7, 430-452.

De Mori, A., Peña Fernández, M., Blunn, G., et al. (2018). 3D printing and electrospinning of composite hydrogels for cartilage and bone tissue engineering. *Polymers (Basel)*, 10(1), 285.

Duarte Campos, D. F., Blaeser, A., Buellesbach, K., Sen, K. S., Xun, W., Tillmann, W., Fischer, H. (2016). Bioprinting organotypic hydrogels with improved mesenchymal stem cell remodeling and mineralization properties for bone tissue engineering. *Adv. Healthc. Mater.*, 5, 1336-1345.

Dupret-Bories, A., Vergez, S., Meresse, T., Brouillet, F., & Bertrand, G. (2018). Contribution of 3D printing to mandibular reconstruction after cancer. European Annals of Otorhinolaryngology. *Head and Neck Diseases*, 135(2), 133-136.

Fielding, G., Bose, S. (2013). SiO_2 and ZnO dopants in three-dimensionally printed tricalcium phosphate bone tissue engineering scaffolds enhance osteogenesis and angiogenesis *in vivo*. *ActaBiomater.*, 9, 9137-9148.

Gao, G., Schilling, A. F., Yonezawa, T., Wang, J., Dai, G., Cui, X. (2014). Bioactive nanoparticles stimulate bone tissue formation in bioprinted three-dimensional scaffold and human mesenchymal stem cells. *Biotechnol. J.,* 9, 1304-1311.

Habibovic, P., de Groot, K. (2007). Osteoinductive biomaterials - properties and relevance in bone repair. *J. Tissue Eng. Regen. Med.,* 1(1), 25-32.

Haleem, A., Javaid, M. (2018). Role of CT and MRI in the design and development of orthopaedic model using additive manufacturing. *Journal of Clinical Orthopaedics and Trauma*, 9(3), 213-217.

Haleem, A., Javaid, M. (2019). Polyether ether ketone (PEEK) and its 3D printed implants applications in the medical field: An overview. *Clinical Epidemiology and Global Health*, 7(4), 571-577.

Haleem, A, Javaid M. (2019c). 3D scanning applications in medical field: a literature-based review. *Clinical Epidemiology and Global Health*, 7(2), 199-210.

Hamlet, S. M, Vaquette C., Shah, A., Hutmacher D. W., Ivanovski, S. (2017). 3-dimensional functionalized polycaprolactone-hyaluronic acid hydrogel constructs for bone tissue engineering. *J. Clin. Periodontol.*, 44, 428-437.

Javaid, M., Haleem, A. (2019a). 4D printing applications in medical field: A brief review. *Clinical Epidemiology and Global Health*, 7(3), 317-321.

Javaid, M., Haleem, A. (2019b). Current status and applications of additive manufacturing in dentistry: A literature-based review. *Journal of Oral Biology and Craniofacial Research*. 9, 179-185.

Kou, P. M., Babensee, J. E. (2011). Macrophage and dendritic cell phenotypic diversity in the context of biomaterials. *J. Biomed. Mater. Res. A.*, 96(1), 239-260.

McCulloch, R. A., Frisoni, T., Kurunskal, V., Maria Donati, D., & Jeys, L. (2021). Computer navigation and 3D printing in the surgical management of bone sarcoma. *Cells*, 10(2), 195.

Moncal, K. K., Aydin, R. S., Abu-Laban, M., Heo, D. N., Rizk, E., Tucker, S. M., Lewis, G. S., Hayes, D., Ozbolat, I. T. (2019). Collagen-infilled 3D printed scaffolds loaded with miR-148b-transfected bone marrow stem cells improve calvarial bone regeneration in rats. *Materials Science and Engineering: C.* 105, 110128.

Nukavarapu, S. P., Kumbar, S., Laurencin, C. (2009). Biodegradable polyphosphazene scaffolds for tissue engineering. *Polyphosphazenes for Biomedical Applications Taylor & Francis group*, 117-138.

Park, J. B. (2011). The use of hydrogels in bone-tissue engineering. *Med. Oral Patol. Oral Cir. Bucal.*, 16(1), e115-e118.

Qasim, M., Chae, D. S., Lee, N. Y. (2019). Advancements and frontiers in nano-based 3D and 4D scaffolds for bone and cartilage tissue engineering. *Int. J. Nanomedicine.*, 14, 4333-4351.

Sa, M. W., Nguyen, B. B., Moriarty, R. A., Kamalitdinov, T., Fisher, J. P., Kim, J. Y. (2018). Fabrication and evaluation of 3D printed BCP scaffolds reinforced with ZrO_2 for bone tissue applications. *Biotechnol. Bioeng.*, 115, 989-999.

Saad, B., Kuboki, Y., Welti, M., Uhlschmid, G. K., Neuen-schwander, P., Suter, U. W. (2000). DegraPol-foam: a degradable and highly porous polyesterurethane foam as a new substrate for bone formation. *Artif. Organs.*, 24(12), 939-945.

Seitz, H., Rieder, W., Irsen, S., Leukers, B., Tille, C. (2005). Three-dimensional printing of porous ceramic scaffolds for bone tissue engineering. *J. Biomed. Mater. Res. B Appl. Biomater.*, 74, 782-788.

Sheller, M. R., Crowther, R. S., Kinney, J. H., Yang, J., Di Jorio, S., Breunig, T., et al. (2004). Repair of rabbit segmental defects with the thrombin peptide, TP508. *J. Orthop. Res.*, 22(5), 1094-1099.

Shen, C., Witek, L., Flores, R. L., Tovar, N., Torroni, A., Coelho, P. G., Young, S. (2020). 3D Printing for Craniofacial Bone Tissue Engineering. *Tissue Engineering Part A*, 26(23-24).

Slaughter, B. V., Khurshid, S. S., Fisher, O. Z., Khadem-hosseini, A., Peppas, N. A. (2009). Hydrogels in regenerative medicine. *Advanced Materials (Deerfield Beach, Fla)*, 21(32-33), 3307-3329.

Tanataweethum, N. (2015). Fabrication of poly-l-lactic acid/dicalcium phosphate dihydrate composite scaffolds with high mechanical strength-implications for bone tissue engineering. *J. Funct. Biomater.*, 6(4), 1036-1053.

Vaishya, R., Vijay, V., Vaish, A., Agarwal, A. K. (2018). Computed tomography-based 3D printed patient-specific blocks for total knee replacement. *J. Clin. Orthop. Trauma*, 9, 254-259.

Witte, T. M. D., Fratila-Apachitei, L. E., Zadpoor, A. A., Peppas, N. A. (2018). Bone tissue engineering via growth factor delivery: from scaffolds to complex matrices. *Regenerative Biomaterials*, 5(4), 197-211.

Chapter 9

Bioprinting of Heart Tissue

Duygu Keser*

Enka Technical School, Kocaeli, Turkey

Abstract

Bioprinting technology is one of the most actual applications in tissue engineering. This technology is a production method that uses 2D, 2.5D, 3D or 4D bioprinters. Living cells, biomaterials, and bioactive molecules are used in this technology. Using bioprinting technology, tissue- or organ-like architectures can be produced from multiple cell types. Additionally, this type of printing process was automated through computer-aided design templates. For example, tracheal splint and aortic valve tissue substitutes can be produced by 3D printing, which was first described by Charles W. Hull in 1986. According to their working principles, there are three types of 3D bioprinters: laser-based, inkjet-based, and extrusion-based bioprinters. In terms of affordability and maneuverability of extrusion-based bioprinting, it is the most powerful 3D printing technology. Two types of ink, organic and inorganic, are used in the 3D printing technique. For instance, while ceramics, metals, and glass-ceramics are inorganic inks, thermoplastics and hydrogels are used as organic inks. Some of the biomaterials used are as follows: cobalt-chrome, titanium, magnesium, and stainless steel. Extrusion-based bioprinters with pneumatic or screw-driven rotational force to move a cellular bioink through a nozzle for cardiac tissue are among the most widely used systems. The need for organ transplants has continuously increased. However, despite this need, unfortunately, no significant increase in the number of donations has been observed. The most important reason for morbidity and mortality are cardiovascular

* Corresponding Author's Email: dukeser@gmail.com.

In: Bioprinting the Human
Editors: Soner Şahin and Kenan Demir
ISBN: 978-1-68507-993-2

diseases. The first remedy to develop heart tissues and heart valves is fabricated using 3D organ biofabrication methodologies, such as bioprinters. Some researchers believe that smart materials and 4D bioprinting techniques will be extremely important for designing soft robotic systems and the architecture of hierarchical, complex, thick, and vascularized tissue structures in the immediate future.

Keywords: bioprinting, heart, biomaterial, bioprinters

Introduction

Copying text or images onto paper with ink is the field of application where printing is most commonly used. Rapid prototyping was introduced to the market as a result of the development and use of three-dimensional (3D) printing technology in the late 1980s (Sirringhaus et al., 2000). Charles W. developed the first 3D printer in 1986, which was introduced by Hull as "Stereolithography" (Hull, 1986). Moroni et al. described "3D printing" on the basis of the printing process appearance that has cell-laden inks (Moroni et al., 2008). Accordingly, in the mentioned additive production technology, a binder jet is directed at a powder bed with the aim of defining a sample. When the solvent's binding to the powder occurs, a small part of the solid material is formed. A novel powder layer is set, and the scaffold is created layer by layer by repeating the said process. The first patent for 3D printing where a binder solution was placed in a powder bed in line with the Computer-Aided Design (CAD) model described by Sachs et al. constitutes the basis for this definition.

The basis for this description was the first patent for 3D printing introduced by Sachs et al. In the said patent, a binder solution was placed in a powder bed following a Computer-Aided Design (CAD) model (Gross et al., 2014). However, 3D printing is expressed as the additive manufacturing process of 3D objects starting from a 3D digital model. For this reason, the locution of 3D printing is still utilized rather than additive manufacturing due to its not being difficult (Kozaniti et al., 2021).

Biological materials are used in this method to produce 3D scaffolds. The development of water-based systems without solvents allows biological materials to be printed directly as 3D tissue scaffolds. Processes can be performed without cells or with cells. 3D bioprinting has been recently used in conjunction with materials science, cell biology, and tissue engineering (Mironov et al., 2009). Bioprinting is a newly developed method that uses new fabrication technologies such as 3D printing or 3D printing of complex tissues/organs to overcome the limitations of traditional tissue engineering techniques (Zhang et al., 2019). In addition, this method is used to control cells in the placement of biomaterials. The fabrication technique is based on the principle of rapid prototyping, which is created by building 3D objects layer by layer by reading the virtually designed data of computer-aided design (CAD) drawings.

The microarchitecture of natural texture is extremely complex due to its 3D environment. Therefore, instead of 2D or 2.5D printing, cells grow, proliferate, and differentiate more similarly to native tissue in 3D environments (Cukierman et al., 2001; Cukierman et al., 2002; Edelman et al., 2005). Furthermore, 3D bioprinters are very suitable for tissue development or regeneration and controlled drug release function integrated into the tissue engineering framework (Cukierman et al., 2001). Tissue substitutes such as the tracheal (airway) splint and aortic valve can be produced with 3D bioprinting technology (Bracci et al., 2013; Duan et al., 2013).

3D bioprinting approaches are biomimicry, self-assembly, and microtissue structures. One of the important problems in printing technology is the incorporation of molten plastics, polymers, and metals into living cells and difficulties in co-pressing with biological materials. Another important problem is that the system is insufficient to replicate biological functions to reproduce the complex microarchitecture of the extracellular matrix (Murphy and Atala, 2016).

3D bioprinters, according to their working principles, have 3 types: laser-based (laser-assisted), inkjet-based, and extrusion-based bioprinters. The most commonly used technique in production is the spin-based bioprinting technique. It is based on distribution using a bioink plastic needle tip in syringes by mechanical or pneumatic force (Hölzl et al., 2016).

Inkjet-Based Bioprinters

Inkjet-based bioprinting applications eject bioink droplets onto a substrate using thermal, acoustic, or electrical energy based on printing layer by layer. The most significant advantage is that the system is cheap and fast (Zhang et al., 2019; Skardal, 2015).

Laser-Based Bioprinting

Laser-based bioprinting applications use the energy of lasers for the purpose of 3D printing. In this method, a laser beam is sent along the "z" axis onto the photocurable bioink that interacts with the light. The final structure is obtained by applying the same process layer by layer. Because the method does not require the use of a needle tip, the cells are not under stress during bioprinting. Therefore, the viability rate for the first time in laser-based bioprinting systems is higher than in needlepoint bioprinting techniques (Zhang et al., 2019; Skardal, 2015).

Extrusion-Based Bioprinters

Extrusion-based bioprinters work on the principle of injecting the bioink contained in a syringe through a needle tip with pneumatic or mechanical force. In bioprinters that use mechanical force, the bioink flowing with the help of a plunger or screw in the syringe flows from the needle tip under the pressure implemented into the syringe in bioprinters using pneumatic force. Extrusion-based bioprinters are the most commonly used bioprinters. The probability of cells being stressed during the printing process is one of the major disadvantages of the method (Zhang et al., 2019; Skardal, 2015).

Owing to 3D printers, layered manufacturing is performed. It is more advantageous in terms of cost and production speed compared to the production with the traditional method. Several parameters are significant when designing or determining the suitability of a skeleton for use in tissue engineering, regardless of the type of tissue. There are some basic requirements to consider before developing intelligent 3D tissue skeletons for tissue engineering and regenerative medicine: mechanical properties, decay rate, porosity, scalability, surface properties, inhibition of immunity and foreign object reaction, bioactivity, etc. (Seal, 2001).

3D bioprinting technology is one of the new applications, providing an alternative solution to problems in some applications of tissue and organ engineering research. 3D bioprinters have different working principles, are capable of producing high-precision 3D structures, have highly variable bioink options, and almost identical structures are obtained in every trial. Due to these advantages, 3D bioprinters have taken a significant place in tissue and organ engineering applications. Tissue engineering tries to overcome the limitations of traditional techniques with the potential advantages of gene therapy and bioprinters (Murphy and Atala, 2014; Chua and Yeong, 2014).

Two types of ink, organic and inorganic, are used in the 3D printing technique. For instance, ceramics, metals, and glass-ceramics are inorganic inks, whereas thermoplastic and hydrogels are used as organic inks. Some of the biomaterials used are cobalt-chrome, titanium, magnesium, and stainless steel. Calcium phosphates, such as brushite, hydroxyapatite, and monetite, belong to ceramics. Calcium oxide, silicon dioxide, sodium oxide, and phosphorus pentoxide belong to glass-ceramic bioglass. Polyglycolic acid (PGA), polylactic acid (PLA), and polycaprolactone (PCL) are some of the most commonly used thermoplastics in the organic category. Hydrogels are divided into synthetic (polyvinyl alcohol—PVA; polyethylene glycol—PEG; or polyacrylic acid—PAA), semi-synthetic (such as derivates of hyaluronic acid, collagen, and elastin), and natural (such as polysaccharides, polynucleotides, and polypeptides) categories (Kampen et al., 2019).

As specified by Moroni et al., it is possible to compose material(s) and biological molecules or cells to formulate a bioink (Moroni et al., 2019). Numerous current reviews have presented a summary of the latest achievements in the bioink area (Han et al., 2019; Güngor-Ozkerim et al., 2018; Jang et al., 2018; Holzl et al., 2016).

Substances, cells, and various biological molecules can be used in a bioink formula (Moroni et al., 2019). Numerous recent reviews have summarized the latest achievements in the area of bioinks (Han et al., 2019; Güngor-Ozkerim et al., 2018; Jang et al., 2018; Holzl et al., 2016). In these papers, natural biomaterial-based bioinks, particularly gelatin, alginate, and fibrin, have been preferred in vascular tissue engineering applications.

While planning a bioink, biological and rheological topics, stability and printability are considered and balanced (Kampan et al., 2019). Furthermore, considering a bioink, crosslinking capabilities, viscosity, and gelation are used as the basic characteristics (Malda, 2013). The bioink characteristics determine the extent of the deviation of the manufactured structure from the design (Kacarevic et al., 2018). For instance, if there is an increasing step in viscosity, this provides better fidelity. However, an increase in shear stress causes cell damage and activates misleading biophysical cues regarding the ECM elasticity and pore properties (Kampan et al., 2019).

The compatibility of the 3D-fabricated structure is related to the rate of transition to the solid state of the bioink after deposition. Due to the reduced gelation time, the solubility of the construct develops after ejection (Kampan et al., 2019). Due to nanoparticles with the innate property of drug delivery, it is possible to improve mechanical and rheological characteristics (Ahlfeld et al., 2017; Baumann et al., 2017). If sodium alginate and human umbilical vein smooth muscle cells are combined and vascular channels are printed by an extrusion-based printer, an increase in proliferation rate and ECM formation are observed (Zhang et al., 2015). According to reports, zigzag vascular tubes were produced by an inkjet-based bioprinter (Xu et al., 2012). After 72h, the apparent amount of fibroblasts was at least 80%. Furthermore, laser bioprinters have been developed to form a vascular-like network. Additionally, there is one more property with regard to improving: the interaction between various cell types (Gruene et al., 2011). There are two categories in terms of cell source: allogeneic and autologous. Human umbilical cord, embryonic stem cells, and cardiomyocytes are included in the allogeneic category. The second category includes induced pluripotent stem cells (iPSCs), adipose stem cells, skeletal stem cells, and bone marrow-derived stem cells (Chaudhuri et al., 2017).

Hitherto, neural engineering, scaffolding tissue production techniques, and many other techniques have been used for functional tissue production (Bracagilia et al., 2017). All these techniques have many advantages, but none of them are 3D bioprinting methods with high precision in cells and the production of 3D organs by placing tissues on top of each other. They do not have such capabilities. Biological patterns produced by bioprinters are highly continuous and stable. In this way, a simulation of the heart's key state with high resolution can be obtained. Additionally, next-generation technology can ensure the exploration of myocardial tissue repair and regeneration in an innovative way (Ong et al., 2018; Ma et al., 2018). Nevertheless, artificial heart muscle tissue is hard to produce due to its multilayered structure. The endothelium of myocardial tissue should be surrounded by layers and fed by blood vessels (Chiu et al., 2011). For these reasons, the production of heart muscle tissues in a laboratory environment is extremely difficult to use for clinical trials (Chiu et al., 2011). However, studies on heart tissue production are extremely important for pathology, cardiotoxicity, and new drug development (Akpek, 2017). The exploration of heart regeneration technology based on 3D bioprinting is still in its early stages. Therefore, it should be studied in a multidisciplinary way. For instance, for a better characterization of the myocardium's physiological complexity and structure, it is necessary to investigate the bioink parameters in the said technology in a continuous manner at chemical and physical levels (Shao, 2020).

During the operation, bioprinting is preferred and plays a critical role in eliminating the difficulty of delivering cells with the least shear stress.

Moreover, it is important that no damage occurs (Roche et al., 2020). There are many reports about bioprinters, bioinks, hydrogels, and some approaches for printing cells into the three-dimensional myocardium (Noor, 2019). Extrusion-based bioprinters that have a pneumatic or screw-driven rotational force to move a cellular bioink through a nozzle for cardiac tissue represent one of the most widely used systems (Puluca et al., 2019).

One of the most important milestones in the field of medicine is organ transplantation. It is the only way that offers more hope for the lives of people who suffer from various diseases that cause end-stage organ failure and death (Kalra and Desousa, 2011). The need for organ transplants has continuously increased. However, despite this need, unfortunately, no significant increase in the number of donations has been observed. For this reason, hundreds of thousands of people lose their lives waiting for transplants every year. This number increases every year. One of the areas where organ transplantation manifests itself as a need the most is heart valve diseases. Heart valve diseases are still one of the most important causes of death in the world (Driessen, 2007). More than 290,000 patients undergo heart valve surgery every year. It is estimated that this number will increase annually to reach 850.000 by 2050 (Balguid et al., 2007; Engelmayr and Rabkin, 2007). For the treatment of heart valve diseases, two types of artificial heart valves are used, mechanical artificial heart valves and bioprosthetic artificial heart valves (Soldian, 2000). The main disadvantage of these two artificial heart valves is that the valves cannot develop with the patient's body after transplantation. This particularly causes serious problems in children, because as children grow, the heart valves have to grow. Children have to undergo surgery again every two to three years and have their heart valves updated with a new model. Additionally, mechanical heart valves are open to infection, inflammation, and thrombosis. Similarly, bioprosthetic heart valves cause thickening and hardening of the heart valves due to calcification, resulting in insufficient closure and therefore leakage (Hoerstrup et al., 2000).

For patients with end-stage heart failure, heart transplantation (HTx) has become a common cure. Due to the development of immunosuppressants, surgical techniques, donor procurement and post-HTx care, there has been a significant reduction in acute allograft rejection. However, long-term survival of allografts has several limitations, such as infection, coronary allograft vasculopathy, rejection, and malignancy (Kim et al., 2018).

In short, cardiovascular diseases are the leading cause of morbidity and mortality worldwide. These diseases cause the deaths of more than 20 million people every year. More than 600,000 cardiovascular surgical procedures are performed each year, which costs approximately $200 billion. Furthermore, the most common cardiovascular diseases are heart tissue diseases that result in heart attacks (Akpek, 2017). Every year, these diseases cause the deaths of more than 17.9 million people, which is about 31% of all deaths around the world (Hert et al., 2018). Furthermore, the healthcare costs of cardiovascular diseases in European countries are estimated at 196 billion euros (Fanourgiakis and Kanoupakis, 2013). More than 80% of CVD death occurs in low- and middle-income countries (Ashna, 2015). Therefore, the necessity to reduce the economic burden cannot be discussed. CVDs involve a large and complex group of diseases, such as peripheral artery disease (PAD), cerebrovascular disease, coronary heart disease (CHD), and rheumatic heart disease. One of the first solutions to this problem is to develop heart valves and heart tissues produced with 3D organ biofabrication methodologies such as bioprinters (Akpek, 2017).

3D printing or bioprinting represents the most successful method, which can be used to partially or completely replace natural organs in the human body, successfully regenerate different organs, blood vessels, and scaffolds (Rathesh et al., 2017). 3D bioprinting technology uses a layer-by-layer overview that provides precise control over biomaterials and cells, which leads to accuracy in architectural construction (Zhang et al., 2019).

Biomaterials, such as natural or synthetic hydrogels or decellularized matrices, are mainly used in 3D printing for the engineering of cardiovascular tissues with the objective of mimicking the dense vascular network that supports the heart tissue. These matrices provide an interconnected porous network, allowing for cell migration, proliferation, and receiving essential nutrients and a sufficient oxygen supply (Zhu and Marchant, 2011) This considers the limitation of the survival distance for cells at a distance of 100-200 μm and less from blood vessels (Muschter et al., 2004).

In bioprinting, collagen and alginate represent the most widely utilized hydrogels after gelatin methacrylate, fibrinogen, and gelatin (França et al., 2004). After printing, cell viability, morphology, and proliferation are significantly influenced by the properties of the chosen bioink (Malda et al., 2013). The difficulty of bioink design is to improve printability and not reduce cell viability at the same time (Kampan et al., 2019). Biomaterial-based hydrogels have cell encapsulation properties. Fibroblasts, endothelial cells, cardiomyocytes, and smooth muscle cells are the primary cell types that integrate cardiac tissue. Furthermore, it is mandatory to perform a computational simulation with the anatomical data and features of a patient to provide an integrated patient-specific bioprinted construct (Kozaniti, 2021).

Problems with organ models and cardiac tissue engineering are faced because of the natural structure of the myocardium. The need to integrate blood vessels limits current approaches suitable for the production of integrated cardiovascular organoids. This need creates additional complexity (Zhang et al., 2016). To produce engineered cardiac tissue and translational applications in medicine, 3-dimensional bioprinting technologies are highly promising despite these problems (Puluca, 2019). Recently, researchers have been exploring higher-level equations of potential 4D bioprinting-based regenerative medicine. In the last 10 years, 3D bioprinting technologies for cardiovascular regeneration and repair have made significant progress, especially to create a holistically engineered heart tissue (HEHT) with long-term contractility for transplantation. In particular, generating HEHT by the 3D bioprinting system is highly dependent on the accurate deposition of a cardiac cell-loaded polymeric bioink in a well-organized way to effectively create the prototypically constructed pathway. These bioprinters are a mechanical construct that redraws the anatomy and pump function of a mammalian heart. Designing the mentioned mechanical operation in a realistic manner has become increasingly profound due to the microscale control advancement of 3D printing technology and cardiac-focused developments of iPSCs and biomaterials (Liu et al., 2021). Researchers working with 3D bioprinting are focusing on strict fitting of an adequate number of functional CMs with a microscale viable scaffold because it is difficult to regenerate and repair damaged or defective hearts. The source of cells applied to the discovery stage can be selective. Their common criterion is the way to provide qualified long-term survival and powerful export of the exquisite bionic body *in vitro* and *in vivo* (Liu et al., 2021) (Correia et al., 2019). The polymer network of the biomaterial that acts as the skeleton and ECM is involved in maintaining the shape of the organizations related to the heart in question. From time to time, it must ensure the release of inner bioactive molecules in a controlled way (Thattaruparambil, 2009). These dynamic factors have to be measured and controlled. The basis for establishing its muscle-like systematic stability must be the appropriate mastery of the protein-cell, cell-cell and cell-ECM interactions that underlie bottom-up heart tissue production (Netto et al., 2019). Today, 3D bioprinting strategies focus on fine-tuning heart-focused engineering examinations before, during, and after bioprinting to fabricate functional cardiac assemblies. There are many studies on cardiac tissue engineering. This indicates that the requirement standards for internal technical specifications can be more stringent in comparison with common approaches (Chen et al., 2008). Researchers have created a new system of multiform paradigmatic methodologies ranging from preparing a bioink to *in situ* biofunction assessment of a 3D engineered HEHT. Due to the inductive analysis of the mentioned classical results, we enumerate leading lines for the standardized and innovative development of highly active cardiac replicates. Furthermore, a good trend reference is provided for a 3D bioprinting engineering roadmap in other organs and tissues (Liu et al., 2021). Recently, studies have been conducted with 4D bioprinters. Some researchers believe that smart materials and 4D bioprinting techniques will be of extreme importance for designing soft robotic systems and the architecture of hierarchical, complex, thick and vascularized tissue structures in the immediate future. Various methodologies used by scientists have obtained a lot of useful information and applications from the structures acquired as a result of the combination of living cells and biomaterials. However, there are fundamental problems in real applications of the obtained cell and noncell biostructures in the dynamic environment of the human body. For this reason, 4D biofabrication has recently emerged, particularly by taking advantage of 3D bioprinters with adding ‘time’ as the 4th dimension. Here, the objects obtained from 3D bioprinting can change their morphology and functionality because of external stimuli such as temperature, pH, ion, or internal ones, i.e., cells and their components. These biostructures, which can adapt to the dynamic environment of the human body, are expected to bring significant advantages in tissue regeneration, drug development, and the treatment of diseases (Akpek et al., 2020). 3D bioprinting represents an additive manufacturing method for the rapid production of numerous complex 3D constructs with certain control in an automated manner. Nevertheless, there are a few drawbacks related to 3D printing. Currently, printed constructions may not completely mimic the hierarchical structure of living tissues with multiple layers. For this reason, 3D bioprinting technology needs time-dependent behavior that can respond to environmental stimuli. Therefore, it may be possible to form multiple layers that can accurately mimic the hierarchical and complex structure of various organ tissues (Ashammakhi et al., 2018). Moreover, another difficulty of 3D bioprinting technology is nonhomogeneous cell encapsulation within the printed constructs because of the low-viscosity bioink. The term bioink is used for cell encapsulated biomaterials. Furthermore, high-viscosity bioinks require higher pressures during printing stages, which adversely affects cell viability because of the increased shear forces during the extrusion process (Li et al., 2016). To eliminate these deficiencies in existing bioinks, many scientists are focusing on designing advanced bioinks with shear thinning and rapidly self-healing characteristics. In this way, the designed bioinks will have easy printability and cell viability. This will hinder mechanical damage-injuring effects on cells. After extrusion, the viscosity increases, resulting in high precision printability (Wilson et al., 2017; Chimene et al., 2016).

Conclusion

Many researchers working in the field of regenerative medicine have recently tried to improve biomimetic architectures with technology. 3D bioprinting is a tissue microenvironment with high complexity, structure-function hierarchy, complex cytoarchitecture, and tissue-specific compositional technology. Moreover, these bioprinters are a leading technology that ensures the production of biomimetic, multiscale, multicellular tissues having mechanical heterogeneity. Despite the limited number of organ donors worldwide, there is a huge demand for organ transplants. Bioprinting represents a potential technology that is capable of solving the said organ shortage crisis completely as a result of producing functional organs. Significant and commendable progress has been made in the area of bioprinting, which can be used as transplantable tissues in regenerative medicine (Vijayavenkataraman et al., 2018).

Bioprinting technology is one of the most effective applications in tissue engineering. Living cells, biomaterials, and bioactive molecules are used in this technology. This technology is a production method utilizing 2D, 2.5D, 3D, or 4D bioprinters (Cukierman et al., 2001; Cukierman et al., 2002; Edelman et al., 2005). Biomedical technology has been reshaped by bioprinting 3D structures that mimic the natural-like extracellular matrix. Bioprinting technology eliminates different inconsistencies related to existing tissue engineering strategies as a result of ensuring an automated and advanced platform for the production of various biomaterials via the accurate deposition of polymers and cells in a pre-designed manner. Nevertheless, there are some problems with various features of the polymers utilized, controlled distribution, viability, and vascularization of cells, etc. Moreover, there are several handicaps associated with the development of 3D scaffolds that prevent the bioprinting of complex structures. Hence, great efforts are made to explore the potential of some natural and synthetic polymers in bioprinting by adjusting their printability and cross-linking properties, biocompatibility, mechanical and thermal characteristics, biodegradability, etc. (Aljohani, 2018).

Using bioprinting technology, tissue or organ-like architectures can be produced from multiple cell types (Noh et al., 2017). Furthermore, this type of printing process was automated through computer-aided design templates. For example, tracheal (airway) splint and aortic valve tissue substitutes can be produced by 3D printing, which was first described by Charles W. Hull in 1986 (Hull, 1986). According to their working principles, 3D bioprinters have three types: laser-based, inkjet-based, and extrusion-based bioprinters (Hölzl et al., 2016). Extrusion-based bioprinting represents the most significant type of 3D bioprinting printing, creating substitute organs due to its maneuverability and affordability. Materials and cells are stacked in layers in a spatially controlled model with the objective of creating living tissues and organs in extrusion-based bioprinting bioinks (Zhang et al., 2021).

With regard to the affordability and maneuverability of extrusion-based bioprinting, it is the most powerful 3D printing type. Two types of ink, organic and inorganic, are used in the 3D printing technique. For instance, ceramics, metals, and glass-ceramics are inorganic inks, whereas thermoplastics and hydrogels are organic inks. Some of the biomaterials used are cobalt-chrome, titanium, magnesium, and stainless steel (Kampen et al., 2019). Extrusion-based bioprinters that have pneumatic or screw-driven rotational force to move a cellular bioink through a nozzle for cardiac tissue represent one of the most widely used systems (Puluca et al., 2019).

The need for organ transplants has continuously increased. However, despite this need, unfortunately, no significant increase has been observed in the number of donations (Driessen, 2007). Cardiovascular diseases are among the main causes of morbidity and death in the world. Every year, more than 20 million people die from these diseases. At the same time, conjectural healthcare expenses for cardiovascular diseases in Europe are €169 billion (Atella et al., 2009). The first remedy to develop heart tissues and heart valves is to fabricate using 3D organ biofabrication methodologies such as bioprinters (Akpek, 2017). Problems with organ models and cardiac tissue engineering are faced because of the natural structure of the myocardium. The need to integrate blood vessels limits current approaches suitable for the production of integrated cardiovascular organoids. This need creates additional complexity (Zhang et al., 2016). To produce engineered cardiac tissue and translational applications in medicine, 3-dimensional bioprinting technologies are highly promising despite these problems (Puluca, 2019). Recently, researchers have been exploring higher-level equations of potential 4D bioprinting-based regenerative medicine. Some researchers believe that smart materials and 4D bioprinting techniques will be extremely important for designing soft robotic systems and the architecture of hierarchical, complex, thick, and vascularized tissue structures in the immediate future (Akpek et al., 2020).

References

Ahlfeld, T., Cidonio, G., Kilian, D., Duin, S., Akkineni, A.R., Dawson, J.I., Yang, S., Lode, A., Oreffo, R.O.C., Gelinsky, M. (2017). Development of a clay based bioink for 3D cell printing for skeletal application. *Biofabrication*, *9*, 034103.

Aljohani, W., Ullah, W.M., Zhang, X., Yang G. (2018). Bioprinting and its applications in tissue engineering and regenerative medicine. *International Journal of Biological Macromolecules*, *107*, 261-275.

Akpek, A. (2017). Three dimensional bioprinting of tissue engineered artificial heart valves by stereolithography. *21st National Biomedical Engineering Meeting (BIYOMUT)*, Istanbul, Turkey.

Akpek, A., Bal, Ö.A., Alarçin, E., Avci, H., Avcı, M. (2020). Recent advances in 4D bioprinting. *Research Journal of Biomedical and Biotechnology*, *1*(1), 20 – 23.

Ashammakhi, N., Ahadian, S., Zengjie, F., Suthiwanich, K., Lorestani, F., Orive, G., Khademhosseini, A. (2018). Advances and future perspectives in 4D bioprinting. *Biotechnology Journal*, *13*(12), 1800148.

Ashna, D.K., Bowry, M.B., Lewey J., DacSagar, B., Dugani, M.D., Choudhry, N.K. (2015). The burden of cardiovascular disease in low- and middle-income countries: epidemiology and management. *Canadian Journal of Cardiology*, *31*(9), 1151-1159.

Atella, A., Brady, A.L., Catapanoc, J.C., Grahame, I.M., Hobbs F.D.R., Leal J.D., Vanuzzoi, M., Paolettil, R. (2009). Bridging science and health policy in cardiovascular disease: focus on lipid management: A report from a session held during the 7th international symposium on multiple risk factors in cardiovascular diseases: prevention and intervention – health policy, in Venice, Italy, on 25 October, 2008. *Atherosclerosis Supplements*, 10(1), 3-21.

Balguid, A., Rubbens, M.P., Mol, A., Bank, R.A., Bogers, A., Kats, J.P., Mol, B.A.J.M., Baaijens, F.P.T., Bouten, C.V.C. (2007). The role of collagen cross links in biomechanical behaviour of human aortic heart valve leaflets - relevance for tissue engineering. *Tissue Eng*, *13*(7), 1501-1511.

Baumann, B., Jungst, T., Stichler, S., Feineis, S., Wiltschka, O., Kuhlmann, M., Linden, M.., Groll, J. (2017). Control of nanoparticle release kinetics from 3D printed hydrogel scaffolds. *Angew. Chem. Int. Ed*, *56*(16), 4623–4628.

Bracaglia, L.G., Smith, B.T., Watson, E., Arumugassaamy, N., Mikos, J., Fisher P. (2017). 3D printing for the design and fabrication of polymer-based gradient scaffolds. *Acta Biomaterialia*, 56, 3-13.

Bracci R., Maccaroni, E., Cascinu, S. (2013). Transient sunitinib resistance in gastro-intestinal stromal tumors, *N. Engl. J. Med*, *368*, 2042–2043.

Chaudhuria, R., Ramachandrana, M., Moharila, P., Harumalania, M., Jaiswal, A. (2017) Biomaterials and cells for cardiac tissue engineering: Current choices. *Materials Science and Engineering: C.*, *79*(1), 950-957.

Chen Q., Haeding, S., Ali, N., Lyon A.R., Boccaccinia A.R. (2008). Biomaterials in cardiac tissue engineering: Ten years of research survey. *Materials Science and Engineering: R: Reports*, 59 (1–6), 1-37.

Chen, Q.Z., Harding, S.E., Nadire N.A., Alexander, R.L, Aldo, R., Boccaccinia, A. (2008). Biomaterials in cardiac tissue engineering: Ten years of research survey. *Materail Science Engineering*, 59, (1–6), 1-37

Chimene, D., Lennox, K. K., Kaunas, R. R., Gaharwar, A. K. (2016). Advanced bioinks for 3D printing: a materials science perspective. *Annals of Biomedical Engineering*, 44 (6), 2090-2102.

Chua S.C.K, Yeong W.Y. (2011). Additive manufacturing-assisted scaffold-based tissue engineering. Innovative Developments. In: *Virtual and Physical Prototyping*, p. 13-14. CRC Press, London.

Cukierman, E., Pankov, R., Stevens, D. R., Yamada, K. M. (2001). Taking cell-matrix adhesions to the third dimension. *Science*, *294*(5547), 1708–1712.

Cukierman, E., Pankov, R., Yamada, K. M. (2002). Cell interactions with threedimensional matrices. *Current Opinion in Cell Biology*, *14*(5), 633–640.

Driessen, J.V.C., Mol, A., Bouten, C.V.C, Baaijens, F.P.T. (2007). Modeling the mechanics of tissue engineered human heart valve leaflets. *J. Biomech*, *40*, 325-334

Duan B., L.A. Hockaday, K.H. Kang, J.T. Butcher (2013). 3D Bioprinting of heterogeneous aortic valve conduits with alginate/gelatin hydrogels, *J. Biomed. Mater. Res. - Part A.*, 101A, 1255–1264.

Edelman, D.B., Keefer E.W. (2005). A cultural renaissance: *In vitro* cell biology embraces three-dimensional context. *Experimental Neurology*, *192*(1), 1–6

Engelmayr, G.C., Rabkin, E., Sutherland, F.W.H., Schoen, F.J., Mayer, J.E., Sacks, M.S. (2005). The independent role of cylic flexure in the early *in vitro* development of an engineered heart valve tissue. *Biomaterials*, *26*, 175-187

Fanourgiakis J., Kanoupakis E. (2014). Catastrophic healthcare expenditure during economic recession in the field of cardiovascular disease. *Expert Review of Pharmacoeconomics & Outcomes Research*, *14*: 1

França, F.S., Santos, M.G., Prestes, J.P., Alcântara, B., Borges, M.F., Pranke, P. (2021). Bioprinting: A promising approach for tissue regeneration, *Bioprinting*, *22*, e00130.

Han, X., Courseaus, J., Khamassi, J., Nottrodt, N., Engelhardt, S., Jacobsen, F., Bierwisch, C., Meyer, W., Walter, T., Weisser, J. (2018). Optimized vascular network by stereolithography for tissue engineered skin. *Int. J. Bioprint*, *4*(2), 134.

Hann, S.Y.; Cui, H.; Esworthy, T.; Miao, S.; Zhou, X.; Lee, S.J.; Fisher, J.P.; Zhang, L.G. Recent advances in 3D printing: Vascular network for tissue and organ regeneration. *Transl. Res.*, *211*, 46–63.

Hert, M., Detraux, J., Psy M., and Vancampfort, D. (2018). The intriguing relationship between coronory heart disease and mental disorders. *Dialogues Clin Neurosci.*, *20*(1), 31–40.

Hoerstrup, S.P., Sodian, R., Daebritz, S., Wang, J., Bacha, E.A., Martin, D.P., Moran, A.M., Guleserian, K.J., Sperling, J.S., Kaushal, S., Vacanti, J.P., Schoen, F.J., Mayer, J.E. (2000). Functional living trileafet heart valves grown *in vitro*. *Circulation*, *102*, 44-49

Hölzl K., S. Lin, L. Tytgat, S. Van Vlierberghe, L. Gu, A. (2016). Bioink properties before, during and after 3D bioprinting. *Biofabrication*, *8*, 3.

Hull, CW. (1986). Apparatus for production of threedimensional objects by stereolithography, *US Patent 4575330*.

Gross, B., Erkal, L.E., Lockwood, S.Y., Chen, C., Spence, D.M. (2014). Evaluation of 3D printing and its potential impact on biotechnology and the chemical sciences. *Analytical Chemistry*, *86*, 7, 3240–3253.

Gruene, M., Pflaum, M., Hess, C., Diamantouros, S., Schlie, S., Deiwick, A., Koch, L., Wilhelmi, M., Jockenhoevel, S., Haverich, A., Chichkov, B. Laser printing of three-dimensional multicellular arrays for studies of cell–cell and cell–environment interactions. *Tissue Engineering Part C. Methods*, *17*, 10.

Gu, Z., Fu, J., Lin H., He Y. (2020). Development of 3D bioprinting: From printing methods to biomedical applications. *Asian Journal of Pharmaceutical Sciences*, 15(5), 529-557.

Gungor-Ozkerim, P.S., Inci, I., Zhang, Y.S., Khademhosseini, A., Dokmeci, M.R. (2018). Bioinks for 3D bioprinting: An overview. *Biomater. Sci. 6*, 915–946

Jang, J., Park, J.Y., Gao, G., Cho, D.W. (2018). Biomaterials-based 3D cell printing for next-generation therapeutics and diagnostics. *Biomaterials*, 156, 88–106

Kalra, G., Desousa, A. (2011). Psychiatric aspects of organ transplantation *Int J Org Transplant Med*, 2(1)

Kampen, K.A., Scheuring, R.G., Terpstra, M.L., Levato, R., Groll, J., Malda, J., Mota, C., Moroni, L. (2019). Biofabrication: From additive manufacturing to bioprinting. in encyclopedia of tissue engineering and regenerative medicine; Reis, R.L., Ed.; Academic Press: Oxford, UK, 41–55.

Kozaniti, F.K., Metsiou, D.N., Manara, A.E., Athanassiou, G., Deligianni, D.D. (2021). Recent advancements in 3D printing and bioprinting methods for cardiovascular tissue engineering bioengineering, *Bioengineering (Basel) 8* (10), 133

Li, Y. C., Zhang, Y. S., Akpek, A., Shin, S. R., Khademhosseini, A. (2016). 4D bioprinting: the nextgeneration technology for biofabrication enabled by stimuliresponsive materials. *Biofabrication*, 9 (1), 012001.

Liu, N., Xing, Y., Yao, B., Zhao, M., Wu, P., Liu, G., Zhuang, D., Haodong, J., Chen, X., He, Y., Huang, S., Ping, Z. (2021). Advances in 3D bioprinting technology for cardiac tissue engineering and regeneration. *Bioactive Materials*, 6, 1388-1401.

Ma, X., Liu, J., Zhu, W. M., Tang, N., Lawrence, C. Yu (2018). 3D bioprinting of functional tissue models for personalized drug screening and *in vitro* disease modeling. *Adv. Drug Deliv. Rev.*, 132, 235-251

Malda, J., Visser, J., Melchels, F.P., Jungst, T., Hennink, W.E., Dhert, W.J., Groll, J., Hutmacher, D.W. (2013). 25th anniversary article: Engineering hydrogels for biofabrication. *Adv. Mater*, *25*, 5011–5028.

Mallis, P., Michalopoulos, E., Pantsios, P., Kozaniti, F., Deligianni, D., Papapanagiotou, A., Stavropoulos, G. C. (2019). Recellularization potential of small diameter vascular grafts derived from human umbilical artery. *Bio-Med Mater. Eng.*, *30*, 61–71.

Mironov, V., Trusk, T., Kasyanov, V., Little, S., Swaja, R., Markwald, R. (2009). Biofabrication: a 21st century manufacturing paradigm. *Biofabrication, 1*(2):022001.
Moroni, L., Wijn, J. R., Blitterswijk C. (2008). Integrating novel technologies to fabricate smart scaffolds. *Journal of Biomaterials Science, Polymer Edition*, 19(5), 543- 572.
Murphy, SV., Atala, A. (2014). 3D bioprinting of tissues and organs. *Nat Biotechnol*, 32(8):773- 85.
Muschler, G.F., Nakamoto, C., Griffifith, L.G. (2004). Engineering principles of clinical cell-based tissue engineering. *JBJS, 86*, 1541–1558.
Neto, M.D, Oliveria, J.F., Mano, J.F. (2019). Microparticles in contact with cells,: from carriers to multifunctial tissue modulators. *Trends Biotechnol*., 37 (9).
Noh, S., Myung, N., Park, M., Kim, S., Zhang, S., Kang H. (2017). 3D bioprinting for tissue engineering. *Clinical Regenerative Medicine in Urology*, 105-123.
Ong C.S., Nam L., Ong K., Krishnan A., Huang, C.Y., Fukunishi, T. (2018). 3D and 4D bioprinting of the myocardium: current approaches, challenges, and future prospects. *BioMed Res. Int*., 2018, ID 6497242
Puluca, N., Lee, S., Doppler, S., Münsterer, A., Dreßen, M, Krane, M, Wu S.M. (2019). bioprinting approaches to engineering vascularized 3D cardiac tissues. *Current Cardiology Reports*, 21, 90.
Ratheesh, G., Venugopa, J.R., Chinappan, A., Ezhilarasu, H., Sadiq, A., Ramakrishna, S. (2017). 3D Fabrication of polymeric scaffolds for regenerative therapy. *ACS Biomater. Sci. Eng*., 3, 7, 1175–1194
Roche, CD., Brereton, R.J.L, Ashton, A.W., Jackson, C., Gentile, C. (2020) .Current challenges in three-dimensional bioprinting heart tissues for cardiac surgery. *European Journal of Cardio-Thoracic Surgery*, 58, (3), 500–510.
Seal, B. (2001). Polymeric biomaterials for tissue and organ regeneration. *Materials Science & Engineering R: Reports*, 34, 147–230.
Shao, L., Gao, Q., Xie, C., Fu, J., Xiang, M., Liu, Z., Xiang, L., He, Y. (2020). Sacrificial microgel-laden bioink-enabled 3D bioprinting of mesoscale pore networks. *Bio-Des. Manuf*., 3, 30–39.
Sirringhaus, H., Kawase, T., Friend, R.H., Shimoda, T., Inbasekaran, M., Wu, W. (2000). Highresolution inkjet printing of all-polymer transistor circuits. *Science*, 290 (5499), 2123-6.
Skardal, A., Atala, A. (2015). Biomaterials for integration with 3-D bioprinting. *Annals of Biomedical Engineering*, 43, 730–746
Sodian, R., Hoerstrup, S.P., Sperling, J.S., Daebritz, S., Martin, D.P., Moran, A.M., Kim, B.S., Schoen, F.J., Vacanti, J.P., Mayer, J.E. (2000). Early *in vivo* experience with tissue engineered trileaflet heart valves. *Circulation*, 102 (2000), 22-29.
Thattaruparambil, R.N., Vaquette, C., Meinert, C., Samuel, I.D., Ivanovski, S. (2009). Optimization of 3D bioprinting of periodontal ligament cells, *Dent Materials*, 35 (12) (2009) 1683-1694.
Vijayavenkataramana, S., Wei-Cheng, Y., Wen Feng, L., Chi-Hwa, W., Jerry Ying, HF. (2018). 3D bioprinting of tissues and organs for regenerative medicine. *Advanced Drug Delivery Reviews*, 132 (296-332).

Wilson, S. A., Cross, L.M., Peak, C. W., Gaharwar, A. K. (2017). Shear-thinning and thermo-reversible nanoengineered inks for 3D bioprinting. *ACS Applied Materials & Interfaces*, 9 (50), 43449-43458.

Xu, C., Chai, W., Huang, Y., Markwald, R.R. (2012). Scaffold-free inkjet printing of three-dimensional zigzag cellular tubes. *Biotechnol*, 109, 12: 3152-3160.

Zhang, B., Gao, L., Ma, L., Luo, Y., Yang, H., Cui, Z. (2019). 3D Bioprinting: A novel avenue for manufacturing tissues and organs. *Engineering*, *5*, 777–794.

Zhang, L., Yang, L. (2015). Anti-inflammatory effects of vinpocetine in atherosclerosis and ischemic stroke: a review of the literature. *Molecules*, 20, 335-347

Zhang S., Vijayavenkataraman S., Lu W.F., Fuh JYH. (2019). A review on the use of computational methods to characterize, design, and optimize tissue engineering scaffolds, with a potential in 3D printing fabrication, *Journal of Biomedical Materials Research, 107*, 5: 1329-1351

Zhang, T., Zijie, Z.W., Xiahou, Z., Wang, X, Zhang, K., Yin, J. (2021). Bioink design for extrusion-based bioprinting, *Applied Materials Today*, 25, 101227.

Zhang, Y.S., Arneria S.B., Shin, S.R., Zhu K., Goli-Malekabadi, Z., Alemana, J., Colosia, C., Businani, F., Erba D.V., Colin B., Shupe, Thomas, Demarchi D, Moretti M., Raponi M, Dokmeci R.M., Atalam A., khademhosseini A. (2016). Bioprinting 3D microfibrous scaffolds for engineering endothelialized myocardium and heart-on-a-chip. *Biomaterials*, 110, 45-59.

Zhu, J.; Marchant, R.E. Design properties of hydrogel tissue-engineering scaffolds (2011). *Expert Rev. Med. Devices*, 8, 607–626.

Chapter 10

3D Bioprinting for Neural Tissue Engineering

Fatih Ciftci[3,4], Askican Hacioglu[5], Sümeyra Ayan[1,6], Soner Sahin, MD[2] and Cem Bulent Ustundag[1,*]

[1]Department of Bioengineering, Yildiz Technical University, Istanbul, Turkey
[2]School of Medicine, Nisantasi University, Istanbul, Turkey
[3]Department of Biomedical Engineering, Fatih Sultan Mehmet Vakif University, Istanbul, Turkey
[4]Technology Transfer Office, Fatih Sultan Mehmet Vakif University, Istanbul, Turkey
[5]Department of Chemistry, University of Helsinki, Helsinki, Finland
[6]Materials Institute, Marmara Research Center, TUBITAK, Kocaeli, Turkey

Abstract

More than a billion people worldwide are thought to suffer from nervous system disorders. Age-related neurodegenerative diseases are also becoming more and more important. The need for neural tissue engineering (NTE) comes from the stubbornness of self-renewal of nerve cells-tissues after neural damage has occurred. Chronic degenerative diseases or traumatic injuries to the nervous system affect the central nervous system (CNS) and peripheral nervous system (PNS) functions. The PNS has a limited number of neural cell regeneration. Demonstrated

[*] Corresponding Author's Email: cbustun@yildiz.edu.tr.

In: Bioprinting the Human
Editors: Soner Şahin and Kenan Demir
ISBN: 978-1-68507-993-2

neurogenesis of CNS stem cells occurs in the hippocampus, subventricular region, and spinal cord (SC). Damage to the central nervous system can lead to stroke, neurodegenerative disorders, trauma, or encephalopathy. Several methods have now been studied to treat CNS damage, including stem cell modifications directly to the injured site, delivering morphogen to the injured area, or for tissue growth of neural, neural stem, or progenitor cells in vitro on 3D scaffolding.

3D inkjet and microjet printing techniques can be used to print neurons with high cell viability.

Neural stem cell (NSC) embryonic stem cells, plumbing cells, adipose tissue, mesenchymal stem cells, etc. are used in NTE. Glioma stem cells were used to create a glioma tumor (brain tumor) model. Differentiation of neural stem cells into alternative types of somatic cells is feasible through some molecules. Therefore, it is convenient for them to be used by bioprinters. The three-dimensional printing of neural tissue with stem cells facilitates research on neurological functions and diseases, as well as drug trials. In addition, in cases of acute brain trauma and chronic degenerative diseases, it will be possible to transfer patient-specific neural cells to the patient. Printing brain tumor cells to form tumor tissue in this way will allow for a more detailed examination of tumor cells that are resistant to chemotherapy drugs. Further development of the bioprinting method may allow the printing of more complex textures. In addition to neural tissues, studies have been performed with three-dimensional bioprinting technology for heart, skin, liver, fat, and muscle tissues. As a result of all the studies, in order to use this technology in patients and obtain more complex tissues, the need to optimize the biomaterials, bioprinter type, and cells to be used has emerged. When current problems are overcome, in the near future, standard organ transplantation practices may be replaced by organs formed from the patient's own stem cells with three-dimensional bioprinting technology. 3D bioprinting can simulate the complexity of our body accurately by using carefully embedded cells and biomaterials based on the required features. This feature analyzes 3D tissue modeling supported using 3D bioprinting technology.

Keywords: neural tissue engineering, 3D bioprinting, neurodegenerative diseases, glioblastoma, disease models

Introduction

The nervous system is made up of the CNS and the PNS. Damage to the human nervous system affects more than a billion people worldwide and has been associated with neurodegenerative diseases, as well as a wide variety of conditions such as diseases of the brain and brain, spine traumatic SCI, and stroke (Hsu & Chen, 2018; Lougiaki et al., 2019; Owens et al., 2015b; Petcu et al., 2018; Sahai & Gogoi, 2019).

Although the central nervous system did not regenerate in one case, there are currently no medical records that improve the CNS. Current therapies generally focus on the orthopedic treatment of unstable vertebrae and ultimately medical treatment and bone preparation. PNS injury management is easier. Current treatments include brain autografts and allografts. However, it has a wide range of problems, such as donor brain dysfunction, malnutrition, poor metabolism, infectious diseases, and immune problems (Hsu & Chen, 2018). Thus, there appears to be a vital need for alternatives designed as an alternative to autograft applications (Ngan et al., 2021; Owens et al., 2015a). Reconstruction of PNS and CNS damage due to the ineffectiveness of current therapies is a constant challenge for psychiatrists and neurobiologists (Sarker et al., 2018).

As a result, innovative strategies for brain tissue repair are developed. Tissue engineering and regenerative brain medicine offer new therapies for cosmetic surgery. This technology uses an external electrical device, called a scaffold, to create a platform on which cells can travel to areas of damaged tissue and repair them. Neural Tissue Engineering (NTE) - 3D skeletal models have proven to be important for simulating the entire microcellular environment and cell-cell interactions (Bedir et al., 2020a).

Pioneering work in this area is recognized and known 3D arrays that are essential for cellular recovery and the direct transformation of the cellular microenvironment, helping to create living tissue from cellular sources. These scaffolds are loaded with cells and/or growth factors to support the formation of new tissues and accelerate cell differentiation. (Chia & Wu, 2015a; X. Cui et al., 2012; Jian et al., 2018a; S. J. Lee et al., 2018a; Li et al., 2018; Yu et al., 2020).

3D printers are frequently used in tissue engineering and NTE, as well as in many areas. The most important development in 3D printing technology has been the use of biocompatible materials and cells. In the technology called the NTE-dimensional bioprinter, biocompatible materials and living cells that can remain and reproduce in these materials are used as ink. The biocompatible material creates a NTE-dimensional model of the organ to be replicated, organ-specific cells proliferate on this skeleton, and the precursor of the organ or tissue is obtained. In recent studies, these methods have been developed and used to produce functional living human 3D tissues and organs with biological and mechanical properties suitable for tissue and organ function (Chia & Wu, 2015b; D. Song et al., 2021; Z. Wang et al., 2021; Yilmaz et al., 2020). Thus, this technology could lead to artificial organ creation and regenerative medicine studies. In this way, an alternative to organ transfer can be developed.

Tissue engineering has become a focus of research in the medical community in search of alternative therapies (Cadena et al., 2021a; H. Cui et al., 2017; Fantini et al., 2019a; Q. Gu et al., 2018; Knowlton et al., 2018a; S. J. Lee et al., 2018a; Matai et al., 2020a; Zhu et al., 2015a). 3D printed tissue models have been shown to be important for cell interaction. Pioneering work in this area includes cells in scaffold-based biofunctional inks, and the desired tissue is printed in 3D by loading into hydrogels, microcarriers, or decellularized matrix components. The scaffold biomaterial creates an environment to develop tissues in a certain way. While encapsulated living cells proliferate taking the shape of the tissue to be printed, the biomaterial degrades over time. In scaffold-less biofunctional inks, living cells are printed directly to mimic embryonic development. In this bioprinting process, cells are first transformed into neotissues. The resulting new tissues are then matured for large-scale production of functional tissues in specific models/patterns. In addition, in vitro studies can offer solutions with 3D bioprinting technology in the treatment of neurological disorders (Jamieson et al., 2021; Kim et al., 2016; Shiju et al., 2020; Yoo et al., 2017a).

In recent years, NTE has made a significant contribution to research efforts to identify appropriate strategies for recovery from neurological diseases and injuries (Cadena et al., 2021a; Knowlton et al., 2018a; S. J. Lee et al., 2018a). At the same time, the physicochemical properties of the NTE system are essential for neuronal function and capacity. NTEs have also been shown to have the potential to model neurological disorders. Following intensive field research, NTE has undergone a wide range of 3D production processes, including soft lithography, microfluidics, and the application of dies along transverse or axial planes for manufacturing (Sharma et al., 2020a; L. G. Zhang & Kaplan, 2016). Recent studies have shown that subterranean tissue production processes are critical for the movement of the complex microenvironment and cellular and neural circuits. (S. J. Lee et al., 2018a).

The need for NTE arises from the difficulty in self-renewal of nerve cell tissue after nerve damage has occurred. There is limited regeneration of neural cells in the PNS (Accardo et al., 2019; K. J. Pollard et al., 2019; Saliba et al., 2018a; Uemura et al., 2011). Adult stem cell neurogenesis in the CNS occurs in the hippocampus, subventricular region (SVZ), and SC (Bedir et al., 2020b;

Koffler et al., 2019a; X. Liu et al., 2021a; Tian & Li, 2020; Xue et al., 2021). The CNS can be damaged by stroke, neurodegenerative diseases, trauma, and/or encephalopathy. The treatment modalities for CNS injuries in recent years are; some methods currently being explored to treat CNS injuries are stem cell implantation immediately entering the site of injury; application of morphogens to the injury site; *in vitro* growth of neural tissue with stem cells; and 3D scaffolding (Girão et al., 2020; Rothenbücher & Martínez-Serrano, 2019; Soman et al., 2012). For PNS, a fractured ligament may be involved, reattached, and reinnervated using grafts or direct the existing nerve through the cord (Iii & Micro, 2006; Saliba et al., 2018b).

Recent research into the production of small cortices known as corticopoiesis and brain cells, also known as brain organoids, is a mechanism that can promote the field of tissue regeneration. The cortical parent of corticopoiesis is muscle tissue that can penetrate deep into the brain (Mahumane et al., 2018).

Brain organoids are 3D human pluripotent stem cells grown in parts of the cerebral cortex, demonstrating the ability to separate and grow tissue directly using neural progenitors (Bae et al., 2021). Another condition that requires the implantation of a foreign body is the use of recording electrodes. The permanent electrode connector is an instrument used to record signals from the cerebral cortex. Research on PNS stimulation in paralyzed and prosthetic patients may improve our knowledge about neural tissue reinnervation in both the PNS and the CNS (Cadena et al., 2021a; H. Cui et al., 2017; Matai et al., 2020a; Restan Perez et al., 2021; Sharma et al., 2020b; Zhu et al., 2015a). This research has the ability to make a difficult aspect of NTE, the functional innervation of neural tissue, more manageable (Aljohani et al., 2018; Jaqueline L. Vieira et al., 2021; Koffler et al., 2019b; X. Liu et al., 2021a).

This study aims to complement existing data in the rapidly growing field of enhanced bioscaffold materials and lab-on-chip systems for NTE application. Specifically, the first part examines the differences used to create NTE models of contrast, shape, and physicochemical properties. The second section discusses the most important data used to treat CNS and PNS damage using NTE scaffolds and lab-on-chip systems. In addition to presenting the latest improvements to the NTE concept, this study describes current constraints and highlights new capabilities and prospects in this field.

Components of Neural Tissue Bioprinting

Bioink is a bioprintable material used in the 3D bioprinting process. Although many biomaterials are used to create tissue damage or disease, biomaterials, living cells that require heat or organic solvents at the time of printing, are not compatible with advanced bioprinting technology (Badhe & Nipate, 2020; Mobaraki et al., 2020a; Oliveira et al., 2019). Bioinks can be divided into two main types: scaffold-free bioinks and scaffold-based bioinks. In scaffold-free bioinks, embryonic growth mimics neoplastic formation. For the formation of large tissues, this method uses tissue spheroids, cell pellets, and tissue strips (Mobaraki et al., 2020b). Scaffold-based bioinks embed cells in support materials such as microcarriers (types of circular cycles that promote cell growth and adhesion; ECMs, decellularized ECMs (dECMs) or exogenous hydrogels. It is selected based on the rate of degradation by the combined cells, which should be based on the design rate of the ECM. Scaffolds promote cell growth, development, and differentiation, while providing chemical and chemical resistance and properties to guide functional tissue assembly. Although scaffold-based bioinks are likely to be effective, the immunosuppression response can be observed in *in vivo* assays, including issues such as product toxicity, disruption of cell-cell interaction, and time required for scaffolding reduction (Benwood et al., 2021).

Bioink selection, which affects cell printing, development, and growth, is one of the most important components in bioprinting. Hydrogels are divided into two major groups of hydrogels: natural and synthetic. Since the goal is to create a biomimetic microenvironment, electronic devices can be modified to contain bioactive molecules, but hydrogels, which are biopolymers, can be very effective (Abelardo, 2018; Knowlton et al., 2018b; Stapenhorst et al., 2021).

The selection of suitable materials for bioink development remains challenging given the need to achieve printability and shape accuracy along with cell survival (Figure 1) (Chopin-Doroteo et al., 2021; Khoshnood & Zamanian, 2020). Important bioink factors to consider include biocompatibility, chemical composition, biodegradability, and mechanical properties. (i.e., compressive modulus, viscosity, and elastic modulus) (de la Vega et al., 2019). For neural tissue applications, bioinks must mimic the native structure of the target NTE, the ECM. In the bioink model studies to be performed on CNS injuries, the work should be developed based on the components of the ECM related to hyaluronic acid in the CNS (S. Song et al., 2022; X. Wang et al., 2012). The elastic modulus (stiffness) of the matrix has an impact on growth, survival, and mobility by affecting cell signaling. Because brain tissue is generally compatible with a stiffness of approximately 0.5 kPa, relatively soft hydrogels with low interfacial tension are used to mimic brain tissue, allowing cells to move along the tissue-implant line (Knowlton et al., 2018a).

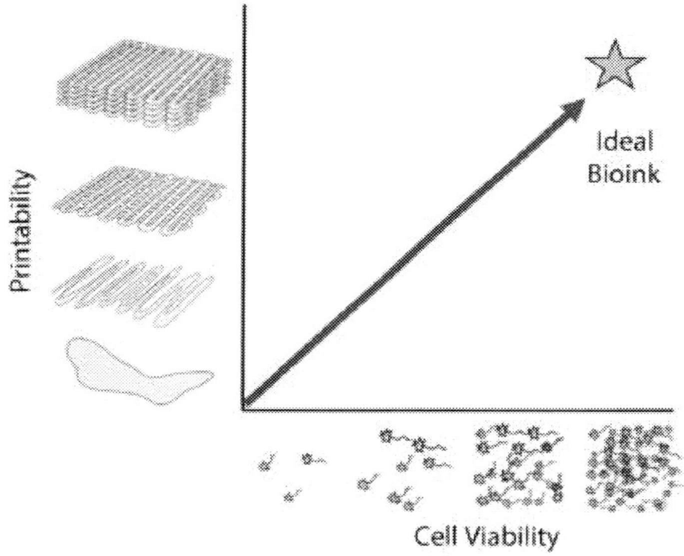

Figure 1. The biofabrication window for advanced biomaterials (Butler et al., 2021a).

Recently, it is known that a 3D biomimetic neural mini-tissue has been produced using a mixture of alginate/agarose and carboxymethyl chitosan as bioinks. The 3D bioscaffold obtained from rapid gelation of bioinks observed the expansion, differentiation, and supporting neuroglia of encapsulated human neural stem cells (Y. Wang et al., 2021a). Fibrin has tunable processes and therapeutic properties and has been linked to a wide range of cells to regulate various tissues, such as the brain (de Melo et al., 2020; C. Lee et al., 2019a). Due to the good cytocompatibility of fibrin, neuronal precursor cells from NTE are dispersed in fibrin bioinks for 3D bioprinting (Y. Wang et al., 2021b).

Butler et al. are investigating the suitability of bioinks for 3D bioprinting, including pure N, O-carboxymethyl chitosan (NOCC), pure agarose and their binary mixtures, and Neuro2A cells in their study. The study showed that to improve the rheological properties, the carboxymethyl chitosan concentration should be increased, while to increase the cellular viability, the agarose concentration should be increased. However, an increase in agarose concentration negatively affects the rheological properties. Therefore, they concluded that they reached a balance in the usage of different materials to obtain the most suitable bioink considering biocompatibility and printability (Butler et al., 2021b).

In the study by Liu et al., they produced laden scaffolds of neural stem cells by 3D bioprinting with a biocompatible bioink consisting of functional chitosan, hyaluronic acid derivatives, and matrigel, against some major challenges such as cumbersome printing process, poor cell viability, and minimal cell-material interaction. They explored their application for *in vivo* SCI repair. They reported that the bioink they developed can gel within 20 seconds and facilitates convenient one-step bioprinting of SC-like structures by spontaneous covalent cross-linking. The scaffolds thus fabricated maintain the viability of high neural stem cells (approximately 95%) and provide a benign microenvironment that facilitates cell-material interactions and neuronal differentiation for optimal neural network formation. The results of the *in vivo* study showed that bioprinted scaffolds promote axon regeneration and reduce glial scar deposition, resulting in a significant locomotor recovery of SCI model rats, which may represent a general and versatile strategy for precision engineering of the CNS and other nervous systems (X. Liu et al., 2021b).

In the Tortorella et al. studies, laminin, one of the main components of brain ECM, is deposited by a laser-assisted bioprinter on a biodegradable scaffold made of poly (lactic-co-glycolic acid) (PLGA), providing chemical indications for the adhesive and differentiation capacity of neural stem cells. Surface roughness and LAB-derived aggregates promote the initial adhesion of neuronal stem cells to the PLGA substrate and influence the formation of clusters and the interconnection between them. The abundance of laminin in the bioprinted structure results in a stronger connection between bioprinted neural tissue structures depending on the morphological analysis (Tortorella et al., 2022).

Bioprinting for the Central Nervous System

Brain Models

Neurological diseases such as Parkinson's disease, Alzheimer's disease, and Alzheimer's disease affect millions of people worldwide (Hopkins, 2015). The weak regenerative capacity of the central nervous system causes serious problems in brain function. In these contexts, appropriate models are needed that allow a deeper understanding and analysis of the pathology and development of neurological diseases. To solve these problems, a great deal of effort has been devoted to creating 3D models of neural tissue *in vitro*, including cell biology-based models (spheres and organoids), neural network mimicry, modeling of neurological diseases, and neurological development (Zhuang, 2018; Dingle, 2015; Jo, 2016; Kato-Negishi, 2013). Despite the great success these studies have achieved, it has been observed that they are insufficient to capture highly viable structures such as the cell-cell and cell-cell-extracellular matrix (ECM) interactions. This is due to its superior ability to simultaneously deposit the cell and the materials used.

There are several important factors to consider when creating neural tissue in vitro. First, there are many neurons and glial cells in different parts of the brain. In addition to neurons, glial cells such as oligodendrocytes, microglia, astrocytes, and pericytes must be determined to provide a fully neural-replicating brain. Second, the ECM is essential for the management of cell behavior. Nerve tissues have unique biophysical properties. Nerve tissue has very low mechanical properties compared to other tissues such as bone, muscle and heart (neonatal tissue 110 Pa and adult tissue <1 kPa) (Benam, 2015).

The materials used to make neural tissue must have similar elasticity patterns to support neurons. These factors are important because most organs and tissues are formed by morphogenetic gradients and must be considered in published data to establish the correct 3D spatial orientation of cells. On the microscopic scale, neurons have a better understanding of key information, including microgrooves, lines, holes, and folds. They have been shown to have important implications for cell migration, differentiation, and neurite development (Li, 2012).

On the macroscopic scale, tissue structure plays an important role in transmitting the necessary signals to the brain. The central nervous system consists mainly of the brain and the SC. The brain is a highly compartmentalized structure with special functions. For example, severe degeneration of the substantia nigra and striatal neurons leads to Parkinson's disease. Alzheimer's disease alters memory abilities and shrinks the hippocampus (D'Avanzo, 2015).

Spinal Cord

SCI continues to be important today due to the high prevalence of SCI in the community, the magnitude of the damage it causes in terms of physical, psychosocial, and economic aspects, and the lack of a universally accepted treatment protocol.

SC is a long artery. Although they show different macrostructures, some differences can be calculated by microstructure. As in the cerebral cortex, aligned fibers are often used to form neural networks and SC. These simple functions can provide a better understanding of tissue formation. The effective pharmacological treatment methods that are being developed reveal the necessity of understanding the pathophysiology of posttraumatic processes (VKH, 1997). Although functional loss is complete in primary or mechanical trauma in patients with SCI, it is rarely the cause of total transsection. In addition, it is known that the damage caused by biochemical and pathological changes in the cord can progress (Faden, 1988). After an acute primary injury, hypoxia occurs in the cord in the early period. After the primary injury to the tissue, a secondary damage period develops in which electrolyte imbalance triggered by hypoxia, neuronal excitation, glutamate release, formation of free radicals, and inflammation are observed (Croft, 1972; Delamarter & Sherman, 1995; Dumont, 2002). In secondary injury, the cascade of triggered events is the result of the activation of endogenous cell death pathways. Despite the promising therapeutic effects of many tested agents, only methylprednisolone therapy has been shown to be effective as a result of large clinical studies (Boyaci, 2014).

Spinal cord injury has not yet been successfully treated. Any damage to nerve and cell bundles that send signals to and from the brain along the human SC can be described as a spinal cord injury. Although damage itself can result from direct injury or bruising of the surrounding vertebrae, the result is often the same: partial or complete loss of sensory and locomotor function below the affected area. Cell-based therapies are the most promising approach for spinal cord injury, though there is no known cure for it. Approaches involve the reconnection of neurons at the injury site for the restoration of nervous functionality, but the regeneration of damaged cells is the biggest problem.

Where neural stem cells were previously implanted at SCI sites, poor viability and uncontrolled differentiation were observed, leading to low therapeutic efficacy. More recent efforts have seen scientists print cell-loaded scaffolds, which can create a favorable microenvironment in which neurons can thrive, but this raises further issues of printability and the initiation of cellular interaction.

Biomimetic 3D scaffolds can be an excellent option for treating brain injuries. 3D scaffolds provide physical support to observe cellular function, allowing the formation of new tissues. Recently, 3D bioprinting technology can control the size and shape of the 3D scaffold and create an attractive mobile phone. 3D bioprinting technology can be used to create biologically complex microstructures. *In vitro* modeling of CNS tissues is critical in the treatment of SCI, particularly for *in vivo* transplantation. Given the potential impact of 3D bioprinting technology on neural studies, this review focuses on 3D bioprinting methods, bioinks, and cells widely used in neural tissue engineering and discusses cutting-edge technological applications of neural tissue bioprinting for SCI repair.

The vital and healthy role of the body is governed by a very complex process called the CNS (Purves et al., 2013; Guillot et al., 2008). Degeneration of CNS structures due to physical or neurological damage often results in loss of brain, axons, and glial support (Lindvall & Kokaia, 2006). The CNS is less able to replace neurons lost due to injury or disease (Zhong & Bellamkonda, 2008). SCI, one of the CNS disorders, damages blood vessels in the brain and other parts of the body. It causes unconsciousness and paralysis below the damage level. There are 11,000 new cases each year in the United States alone, and approximately 450,000 cases are associated with SCI (Qian et al., 2005; Baptiste & Fehlings, 2006a). Car accidents, collisions, falls, and sports injuries account for most injuries (Sekhon & Fehlings, 2001). SCI affects the quality of life of patients, burdens the family and has implications for global health (Venugopal et al., 2017). One of the current treatments for SCI is an overdose of methylprednisolone to reduce the risk of secondary injury (Cheung et al., 2015). However, this treatment is not reliable, as it has many side effects, such as sepsis, ulcers, abdominal bleeding, and pneumonia. Moreover, there is only mild psychiatric treatment (L. J. W. Liu et al., 2020; Z. Liu et al., 2019). Other therapies for spinal fusion include spinal stabilization, reduction of decompression, and multiple therapies, as well as surgery for hypothermia and rehabilitation (Baptiste & Fehlings, 2006b). Despite improvements in various therapies, success in the treatment of neurodegenerative diseases and remodeling of the whole brain remains in infants (Yoo et al., 2017b; Zhu et al., 2015b).

Recent advances in nanotechnology and tissue engineering have provided innovative approaches for the treatment of CNS diseases. Neural tissue engineering focuses on improving the environment necessary to repair and repair functional tissues by connecting cells with biomimetic scaffolds. Physical support for whole-brain processing is provided by three-dimensional (3D) scaffolds and scaffold-like materials (Zhu et al., 2015a; Cunha et al., 2011). This promotes tissue regeneration and the regeneration of new tissue to support cell function (Subramanian et al., 2009a).

An ideal scaffold for neural tissue engineering should follow the following:

a. Biocompatibility is an important tool that allows scaffolds to enhance cell adhesion, proliferation, and differentiation without antibacterial and cytotoxic properties.
b. Biodegradability is essential for the degradation of the scaffold at a cost similar to the connective tissue and the removal of the scaffold from the system.
c. Neurotransmission is based on the efficiency generated by the synapses. Electroencephalography can promote neurite outgrowth and brain regeneration.
d. The skeletal system must have a repair kit to prevent stress on the wound site or breakage during regular use.
e. The interconnected porous scaffolds mimic the extracellular matrix (ECM) of natural tissues to provide vascularization, cell dispersal, elimination, and nutrient exchange (Hill, 2009; Subramanian et al., 2009b).

Various methods such as oil foaming, melt casting, electrospinning, and phase separation have been used to create 3D supports from synthetic and natural polymers (Cheng et al., 2018; Liao et al., 2004). However, this scaffold design process does not control the shape of the scaffold or the channel structure and the pore size of the scaffold. In addition, these techniques do not allow the manufacture of hand scaffolds due to the need for labor.

Recently, 3D bioprinting methods have been proposed to control the size and shape of 3D scaffolds and design cellular scaffolds (Bharadwaj et al., 2021; Cornelissen et al., 2017; B. K. Gu et al., 2016). 3D printing was first described by Charles W. Hull in 1986 (Kruth et al., 1998). 3D bioprinting, also known as additive manufacturing (AM), is the printing of cells, development, and various biomaterials in a multilayer rapid prototyping (RP) system. These processes allow the formation of biological processes close to tissues/organs (Haring et al., 2017). 3D bioprinting uses 3D modeling services (such as computer-aided design (CAD) or computed tomography (CT) images) to create 3D objects or gel-like objects. Typically, a 3D bioprinting system consists of X, Y, and Z-axis actuators, a 3D modeling program, a computer, and a bioprinting/ink source. Start by designing using a CAD or CT diagram. The 3D scaffold structures are then developed using bioprinting equipment connected to a computer (Wong & Hernandez, 2012). Bioink is an important part of 3D bioprinting. Bioinks contain biomaterials that can be used to encapsulate cells and bring together biomolecules. Before printing, attention should be paid to the essential properties of bioinks, such as cross-linking, viscosity, and gelation. These products affect print quality, morphology, cell viability, and proliferation (Malda et al., 2013). According to the principles of processing, extrusion, inkjet, and laser-assisted (X. Wang et al., 2007). In this technology, extrusion bioprinting can create large 3D models using cell-laden hydrogels. Inkjet bioprinting is commonly used in industrial two-dimensional (2D) printers to print liquids containing cells for rapid small-scale production (Hendriks et al., 2015). Laser-assisted bioprinting can use lasers as energy to create high resolution patterns (Du, 2018; Ozbolat & Hospodiuk, 2016; Peng et al., 2017). However, this technique has significant advantages and limitations in the design of structures such as the neural scaffolds mentioned above.

Nerves

PNS is a disease usually caused by a direct injury (Houschyar et al., 2016). Although peripheral arteries do not pose a risk to life, they affect more than a million people worldwide each year and make their lives miserable, including loss of hearing, speech, and movement, paralysis of the brain, and muscle atrophy (Subramanian et al., 2011). In addition to this, the self-healing capacity of peripheral arteries is limited, affecting the age of the patient and the process of injury, especially the similarity of cerebral palsy arteries (Fairbanks et al., 2019). After rupture of the peripheral arteries, the two terminal stumps contract separately. When the distal stump loses nutrients from the nerves of the body, the ridges and myelin degenerate and eventually disappear and relative degeneration returns. If surgery can be performed in time to suture the broken bone to the right, it will promote axonal regeneration and help repair the artery by reaching the correct position. (Dent et al., 2011). Current treatment is surgical resection, which uses the muscle without neural tube sutures. However, if the duration is longer than 5 months, the suture cannot be performed. Autologous brain transplants are the popular model in these cases, but this procedure requires at least two surgeries due to healthy blood vessels and can lead to neuroma recurrence, limited to the brain (Heneka et al., 2010a). Based on the observations above, surgical suturing and autologous nerve transplantation have certain limitations. For this reason, people are looking for solutions through NTE that provide exogenous changes in the connection of blood vessels.

One of the goals of tissue engineering is to create mutations in malignant tissues (Heneka et al., 2010b). In general, scaffolds that provide 3D migration support for cell adhesion, migration, and growth, as well as chemical carriers, are needed (Salles et al., 2018; L. Zhang et al., 2005). Moreover, neural tissue-engineered scaffolds can support neural reconstruction in long-term neural defects up to more than 4 cm in length, providing high precision and microarchitecture (Panigada et al., 2013).

An ideal NTE scaffold can follow the design and structure of the ECM to support cellular tissue proliferation, adhesion, proliferation, differentiation, and formation (Hsu & Chen, 2018). The microgrooves also function to regulate blood vessel growth, such as connecting blood vessels to help repair the brain (Jian et al., 2018b; S. J. Lee et al., 2018b). In studies (Zhu et al., 2015a), a neural channel with four hard-structured microchannels was published. After placing a 3D printed catheter on the amputated sciatic nerve in mice, we found that the regenerated artery splits into four branches at the proximal end and connects to the artery at the distal end, allowing the brain to show positive engagement. This shows that the packaging design model can simulate brain direction and development (Ning et al., 2018a, 2019, 2021a). In the actual situation, the scaffold structure should be designed in a way that damages the hull ships to avoid obstruction of the ship and to follow the instructions of the ship. The high resolution of 3D printers can easily meet the precision and complexity required for neural scaffolds. Neural scaffolds require reprocessing of local vessels and different materials have different tensile strengths. The maximum tensile strength of the normal sciatic and acellular nerve in mice is known from the data of 2.7 and 1.4 MPa (Ning et al., 2018b, 2021b). Therefore, if neural scaffolds are to be planted in mice for animal experiments, their equipment should reach this level. Similarly, when scaffolds are planted in patients, they should first be tested for their ability to resist sensitive and resistive tensile, compressive, and shear forces (Dixon et al., 2018).

Neural scaffolds are believed to be biocompatible and have minimal cytotoxicity and inflammatory responses in the body. They should provide the best cellular sites that facilitate cell adhesion, growth, development, and natural formation to promote the formation and function of damaged blood vessels (Cadena et al., 2021b; Fantini et al., 2019b; S. J. Lee et al., 2018a; Matai et al., 2020b; Zhu et al., 2015a). It depends on the choice of materials and bioactive molecules for neural tissue engineering. Moreover, since one of the most important functions of the neural scaffold is to transmit electricity, it is believed that the best neural scaffold has growth of electrical conduction and cell migration in addition to supporting the body. Nerves that support brain regeneration (H. Cui et al., 2017).

Bioprinted Disease Models for Neural Tissue

Glioblastoma Models

Glioblastoma is one of the most fatal malignant tumors with intractable characteristics. Although 3,19 cases per 100,000 people were reported annually in the US, the incidence is increasing due to the aging population with a 5-year survival rate of 4,7% (Alexander & Cloughesy, 2017; Thakkar et al., 2014). Current treatment strategies involve tumor removal surgery, chemotherapy with DNA alkylating agents, and radiotherapy (Tan et al., 2018). However, the survival rate after diagnosis is less than 2 years (Witthayanuwat et al., 2018).

Treatment of glioblastoma depends on tumor heterogeneity resulting from genetic abnormalities, epigenetic topographic changes, transcriptional dysregulation, microenvironmental cues, and development (Rybin et al., 2021). These features cause variations between different patient tumors. Researchers have recently made a major effort to overcome the heterogeneity issue and develop models of glioblastoma disease to reduce the complexity of the disease.

Glioblastoma cell lines have been available since the end of the 1960s (Pontén & Macintyre, 1968). Since the discovery of the use of glioma stem cells, which can derive models more similar to those of patient tumors, glioma stem cells are commonly used to model brain cancer. (J. Lee et al., 2006). They can be easily isolated from patients and grown in a culture medium using the same growth factors of neural stem cells such as EGF and FGF2 (Azzarelli, 2020; S. M. Pollard et al., 2009). Glioma stem cells can be cultured using 2D and 3D culture methods; however, there are several limitations. For 2D culture in serum, glioma stem cells lose their phenotypic characteristics and observed morphology changes (J. Lee et al., 2006). For the 3D culture of glioma stem cells, the main limitation is obviously the homogeneity of the cultured cells. They lack the ability to reproduce the complex, cellular, and environmental interactions of tumors. Therefore, organoid-based models have been developed (Rybin et al., 2021).

There are 4 different disease model approaches considered to be significant for mimicking glioblastoma:

1. Patient-derived xenograft tumoroids
2. Neoplastic cerebral organoids (NeoCOR)
3. Glioblastoma cerebral organoids (GLICO)
4. Bioprinted Models.

The type of patient-derived xenograft tumor developed by Hubert et al. More bacterial models with different cell types (Hubert et al., 2016). They formed a matrix-supported organoid with patient-derived cancer cells using Matrigel. Glioblastoma tumoroids can be cultured *in vitro* in Matrigel for extended periods with this method. These tumoroids were able to show the features of glioblastomic tissue, including hypoxic gradients, radiation resistance, cellular morphology, and spatial distribution. Jacob et al. improved this model without using Matrigel with a decrease in the time needed (Jacob et al., 2020). They also developed a protocol for the cryopreservation of glioblastoma organoids. Even if they were able to reduce the time frame to form an organoid disease model with this approach, testing personalized therapies for the treatment of glioblastoma is not possible due to the limited therapeutic window. In addition, patient-derived xenografts are not sufficient to mimic the heterogenic tumor environment because of the absence of normal brain tissues, vasculature, and limited immune cell presence (Azzarelli, 2020; Orcheston-Findlay et al., 2021; Rybin et al., 2021).

In 2018, two research teams worked on processes related to brain organoid engineering to cause glioblastoma. (Bian et al., 2019; Ogawa et al., 2018). Neoplastic cerebral organoids (NeoCORs) term annotated by Bian et al. In this approach, oncogenic mutations for initiating tumorigenesis in the iPSC-derived brain organoids created via CRISPR-based genome editing tools. Tumor tracking in these procedures is easily possible with fluorescent markers. The crucial progression of NeoCORs is the ability to make normal cerebral organoids that have tumor formations. That brings the opportunity to study early-stage tumorigenesis and brain-tumor interactions. Although these unique features, NeoCORs have to be studied further to understand how good their ability is to mimic the heterogenic structure of the glioblastoma tumor environment. CRISPR-based mutations are limited either, which limits the variation in mutations to study different types of tumors (Rybin et al., 2021).

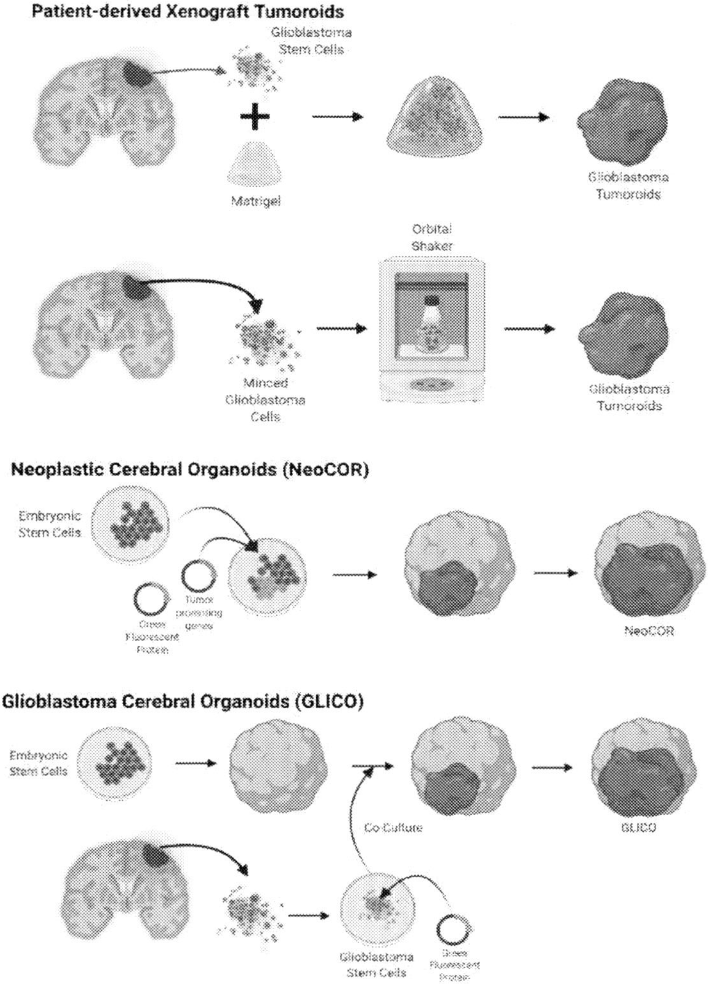

Figure 2. Three-dimensional disease models for glioblastoma.
Created with Biorender.com.

Glioblastoma cerebral organoids (GLICO) are developed by Linkous et al., improving NeoCORs by coculture of patient-derived glioblastoma stem cells and brain organoids derived from iPSC (Linkous et al., 2019). With their approach, the patient-specific formation of glioblastoma can be observed.

They basically combine the advantages of tumoroids and NeoCORs. However, GLICO models are observed to have similar disadvantages of tumoroids, with the formation of no vasculature and the limited presence of immune cells (Rybin et al., 2021).

3D bioprinting can be used to develop custom disease models that meet patient-specific anatomic differences, which is crucial to mimicking the uniqueness of glioblastoma. Cell interactions with ECM component interactions can also be studied with bioprinted models. A shorter time frame is possible to study treatment strategies compared to the other approaches mentioned above. Furthermore, it may be possible to fabricate a vasculature structure with heterogeneity within glioblastoma models (Tang et al., 2021; X. Wang et al., 2021).

A study in 2019 showed the precision of a bioprinted glioblastoma model for drug screening by comparing the failure of a novel treatment method within a 2D cell culture (C. Lee et al., 2019b). A fibrin-based bioink was used and increased expression of glioblastoma stem cell markers was observed. In another study, a drug screening procedure was facilitated with bioprinted glioblastoma organoids that were printed with a new immersion bioprinting method (Maloney et al., 2020).

A study focused on a bioprinting technique for printing low-viscous bioinks with a supporting bath and tried to mimic the conductive environment of brain tissue with a bioink composed of neuroblastoma cells, carbon nanotubes, and nanocrystalline cellulose (Bordoni et al., 2020). Better differentiation aspects were observed within bioprinted structures printed with conductive bioinks.

Microfluidic models are promising for studying BBB interactions and can be called glioblastoma-on-chip approaches (DePalma et al., 2022; Logun et al., 2018). In one study, a patient-specific tumor-on-chip model has been developed with bioprinting dECM components, patient glioblastoma cells, and vascular endothelial cells in a hierarchy (Yi et al., 2019). This hierarchy involves printing vascular cells on the outer side of cancer cells, mimicking one of the most crucial pathological features of glioblastoma (Azzarelli, 2020). This approach was able to show hypoxic features within the printed tumor. Also, the procedure takes 1-2 weeks, which can be considered as an important advantage.

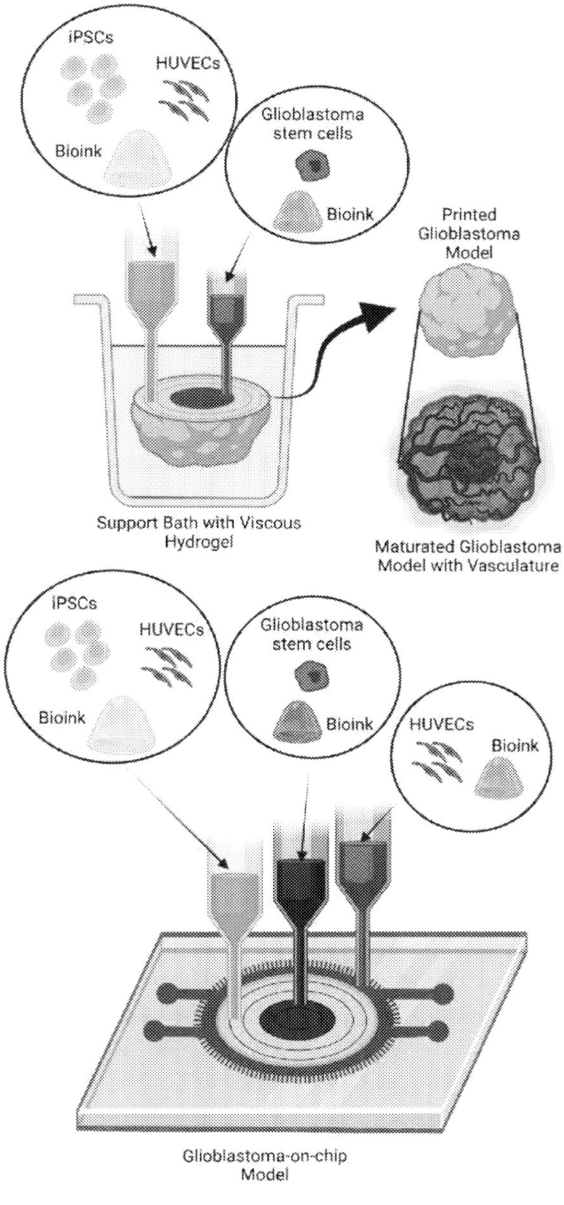

Figure 3. Three-dimensional bioprinted disease model approaches for glioblastoma. Created with Biorender.com.

Silvani et al. studied another tumor-on-chip approach, especially focusing on the permeability of the blood-brain barrier (BBB) of a glioblastoma tumor environment (Silvani et al., 2021). They also performed experiments under simulated microgravity conditions to understand the postoperation conditions, which involve mechanical unloading. As a result, they observed significant differences in blood accumulation and BBB permeability with changing gravitational forces.

Neurodegenerative Disease Models

Due to the aging population, the overcoming neurodegenerative diseases has become a more important challenge today. There is no known cure for neurodegenerative diseases such as Alzheimer's disease, Parkinson's disease, or Huntington's disease. A better understanding of the mechanisms of these diseases is urgently needed to develop better treatment strategies and identify effective pharmacological molecules (Knowlton et al., 2018c).

Animal models have been widely used to understand the mechanisms associated with neurodegeneration. Rodent-based, fish-based, and insect-based animal models have provided essential pathophysiological insights. However, these animal models do not have the ability to fully mimic human diseases with time-consuming procedures (Dawson et al., 2018).

Since iPSCs have been developed and advancements provided in 2D, 3D cell culture methods have been established to form neural tissue lines, *in vitro* neurodegenerative disease models are considered better alternatives due to shorter time frames and better recapitulation capacities of human tissues (Rivetti di Val Cervo et al., 2021; Slanzi et al., 2020). Therefore, 3D bioprinted models are emerging as promising candidates for brain tissue construction, with the objective of better understanding the underlying mechanisms of neurodegenerative diseases. A recent study shows the advantages of 3D bioprinted Alzheimer's disease models by comparing them with 2D and 3D disease models (Y. Zhang et al., 2022). In the study by Zhang et al., better self-renewal capacity and long-term cell viability of neural tissues are observed, as well as increased amyloid-β expression that proves that the bioprinted model is a great candidate for Alzheimer's disease. As research progresses, bioprinted models for neurodegenerative diseases will be the best candidate for understanding the mechanisms and drug development studies.

Conclusion

Three-dimensional bioprinting is a very attractive biofabrication method for producing novel solutions for neural tissue engineering applications. It has demonstrated a high therapeutic capacity to regenerate nerves, SC, and degenerated brain tissues in the literature. Bioprinted minibrains and 3D printed brain-on-chip approaches are also observed to be the best candidates for expanding the knowledge about the pathophysiological mechanisms of neurodegenerative diseases and brain cancer. The high mimicry potential of bioprinted neural tissues makes them the best candidates for creating disease models on glioblastoma and neurodegenerative diseases. 3D bioprinting provides spatial deposition control to create complex architectures that can be designed biomimically. Besides its potential, there should be further studies to recapitulate brain tissues, nervous replicates, and SCs ultimately.

Better bioink candidates should be developed to form more complex architectures due to the low viscosities of current bioink materials. Usually, for the printing of complex structures, bioprinting is performed in a supporting bath. This limits perfect spatial control due to the residual viscous materials of the dissolved support gels. The use of conductive components in bioink formulations is another trend, especially for regenerative approaches. However, safer alternatives should be studied to decrease the toxic and accumulative effects of the currently used materials, such as carbon nanotubes.

Second, iPSC technology should be developed to create different disease models and types of glioblastoma. Bioprinting methods that involve cocultured cell spheroids can be further studied with a bottom-up approach. Another advancement could be in post-printing procedures, which may ultimately lead to mini-systems. A significant step with bioprinted organ-on-chip devices has been made in this manner. However, the biomimicry focus of this biofabrication method will eventually lead to the most complex architectures, and even systems. Furthermore, personalized treatments with patient-specific raw materials will be able to be efficiently enabled by bioprinting disease models and tissue constructs with regenerative capacities.

References

Abelardo, E. (2018). Synthetic material bioinks. *3D Bioprinting for Reconstructive Surgery: Techniques and Applications, 2018,* 137-144. https://doi.org/10.1016/B978-0-08-101103-4.00009-0.

Accardo, A., Cirillo, C., Lionnet, S., Vieu, C., & Loubinoux, I. (2019). Interfacing cells with microengineered scaffolds for neural tissue reconstruction. *Brain Research Bulletin, 152,* 202-211. https://doi.org/10.1016/j.brainresbull.2019.07.020.

Alexander, B. M., & Cloughesy, T. F. (2017). Adult glioblastoma. *Journal of Clinical Oncology*, *35*(21), 2402–2409. https://doi.org/10.1200/JCO.2017.73.0119.

Aljohani, W., Ullah, M. W., Zhang, X., & Yang, G. (2018). Bioprinting and its applications in tissue engineering and regenerative medicine. *International Journal of Biological Macromolecules*, *107*(Part A), 261-275. https://doi.org/10.1016/j.ijbiomac.2017.08.171.

Azzarelli, R. (2020). Organoid Models of Glioblastoma to Study Brain Tumor Stem Cells. *Frontiers in Cell and Developmental Biology*, *8*(April), 1–9. https://doi.org/10.3389/fcell.2020.00220.

Badhe, R. V., & Nipate, S. S. (2020). Cellulosic materials as bioinks for 3D printing applications. In *Advanced 3D-Printed Systems and Nanosystems for Drug Delivery and Tissue Engineering* (pp.109-137*).* https://doi.org/10.1016/b978-0-12-818471-4.00005-4.

Bae, M., Hwang, D. W., Ko, M. K., Jin, Y., Shin, W. J., Park, W., Chae, S., Lee, H. J., Jang, J., Yi, H. G., Lee, D. S., & Cho, D. W. (2021). Neural stem cell delivery using brain-derived tissue-specific bioink for recovering from traumatic brain injury. *Biofabrication*. *13*(4). https://doi.org/10.1088/1758-5090/ac293f.

Baptiste, D. C., & Fehlings, M. G. (2006a). Pharmacological approaches to repair the injured spinal cord. *Journal of Neurotrauma, 23*(3-4):318-334. https://doi.org/10.1089/neu.2006.23.318.

Baptiste, D. C., & Fehlings, M. G. (2006b). Pharmacological approaches to repair the injured spinal cord. *Journal of Neurotrauma, 23*(3-4):318-334. https://doi.org/10.1089/neu.2006.23.318.

Bedir, T., Ulag, S., Ustundag, C. B., & Gunduz, O. (2020a). 3D bioprinting applications in neural tissue engineering for spinal cord injury repair. *Materials Science and Engineering C*., *110*, 110741. https://doi.org/10.1016/j.msec.2020.110741.

Bedir, T., Ulag, S., Ustundag, C. B., & Gunduz, O. (2020b). 3D bioprinting applications in neural tissue engineering for spinal cord injury repair. *Materials Science and Engineering C*., *110*, 110741. https://doi.org/10.1016/j.msec.2020.110741.

Benwood, C., Chrenek, J., Kirsch, R. L., Masri, N. Z., Richards, H., Teetzen, K., & Willerth, S. M. (2021). Natural biomaterials and their use as bioinks for printing tissues. *Bioengineering, 8*(2), 27. https://doi.org/10.3390/bioengineering8020027.

Bharadwaj, T., Thomas, A., & Verma, D. (2021). Bioprinting. *Applications of 3D printing in Biomedical Engineering,* 45-96. https://doi.org/10.1007/978-981-33-6888-0_3.

Bian, S., Repic, M., Guo, Z., Kavirayani, A., & Burkard, T. (2019). Genetically engineered cerebral organoids model brain tumour formation. *Nat Methods, 15*(8), 631–639. https://doi.org/10.1038/s41592-018-0070-7.

Bordoni, M., Karabulut, E., Kuzmenko, V., Fantini, V., Pansarasa, O., Cereda, C., & Gatenholm, P. (2020). 3D printed conductive nanocellulose scaffolds for the differentiation of human neuroblastoma cells. *Cells*, *9*(3). https://doi.org/10.3390/cells9030682.

Butler, H. M., Naseri, E., MacDonald, D. S., Tasker, R. A., & Ahmadi, A. (2021a). Investigation of rheology, printability, and biocompatibility of N,O-carboxymethyl chitosan and agarose bioinks for 3D bioprinting of neuron cells. *Materialia, 18,* 101169. https://doi.org/10.1016/j.mtla.2021.101169.

Butler, H. M., Naseri, E., MacDonald, D. S., Tasker, R. A., & Ahmadi, A. (2021b). Investigation of rheology, printability, and biocompatibility of N,O-carboxymethyl chitosan and agarose bioinks for 3D bioprinting of neuron cells. *Materialia, 18,* 101169. https://doi.org/10.1016/j.mtla.2021.101169.

Cadena, M., Ning, L., King, A., Hwang, B., Jin, L., Serpooshan, V., & Sloan, S. A. (2021a). 3D Bioprinting of Neural Tissues. *Advanced Healthcare Materials, 10*(15), 2001600. https://doi.org/10.1002/adhm.202001600.

Cadena, M., Ning, L., King, A., Hwang, B., Jin, L., Serpooshan, V., & Sloan, S. A. (2021b). 3D Bioprinting of Neural Tissues. *Advanced Healthcare Materials, 10*(15), 2001600. https://doi.org/10.1002/adhm.202001600.

Cheng, T., Qu, H., Zhang, G., & Zhang, X. (2018). Osteogenic and antibacterial properties of vancomycin-laden mesoporous bioglass/PLGA composite scaffolds for bone regeneration in infected bone defects. *Artificial Cells, Nanomedicine and Biotechnology, 46*(8):1935-1947. https://doi.org/10.1080/21691401.2017.1396997.

Cheung, V., Hoshide, R., Bansal, V., Kasper, E., & Chen, C. (2015). Methylprednisolone in the management of spinal cord injuries: Lessons from randomized, controlled trials. *Surgical Neurology International, 6:*142. https://doi.org/10.4103/2152-7806.163452.

Chia, H. N., & Wu, B. M. (2015a). Recent advances in 3D printing of biomaterials. *Journal of Biological Engineering, 9,* 4. https://doi.org/10.1186/s13036-015-0001-4.

Chia, H. N., & Wu, B. M. (2015b). Recent advances in 3D printing of biomaterials. *Journal of Biological Engineering, 9,* 4. https://doi.org/10.1186/s13036-015-0001-4.

Chopin-Doroteo, M., Mandujano-Tinoco, E. A., & Krötzsch, E. (2021). Tailoring of the rheological properties of bioinks to improve bioprinting and bioassembly for tissue replacement. *Biochimica et Biophysica Acta - General Subjects, 1865*(2), 129782. https://doi.org/10.1016/j.bbagen.2020.129782.

Cornelissen, D. J., Faulkner-Jones, A., & Shu, W. (2017). Current developments in 3D bioprinting for tissue engineering. *Current Opinion in Biomedical Engineering.* https://doi.org/10.1016/j.cobme.2017.05.004.

Cui, H., Nowicki, M., Fisher, J. P., & Zhang, L. G. (2017). 3D bioprinting for organ regeneration. *Advanced Healthcare Materials, 6*(1), 1601118. https://doi.org/10.1002/adhm.201601118.

Cui, X., Boland, T., D.D'Lima, D., & K. Lotz, M. (2012). Thermal inkjet printing in tissue engineering and regenerative medicine. *Recent Patents on Drug Delivery & Formulation, 6*(2), 149–155. https://doi.org/10.2174/187221112800672949.

Cunha, C., Panseri, S., & Antonini, S. (2011). Emerging nanotechnology approaches in tissue engineering for peripheral nerve regeneration. *Nanomedicine: Nanotechnology, Biology, and Medicine, 7*(1), 50-9. https://doi.org/10.1016/j.nano.2010.07.004.

Dawson, T. M., Golde, T. E., & Lagier-Tourenne, C. (2018). Animal models of neurodegenerative diseases. *Nature Neuroscience, 21*(10), 1370–1379. https://doi.org/10.1038/s41593-018-0236-8.

de la Vega, L., Lee, C., Sharma, R., Amereh, M., & Willerth, S. M. (2019). 3D bioprinting models of neural tissues: The current state of the field and future directions. *Brain Research Bulletin, 150,* 240-249. https://doi.org/10.1016/j.brainresbull.2019.06.007.

de Melo, B. A. G., Jodat, Y. A., Cruz, E. M., Benincasa, J. C., Shin, S. R., & Porcionatto, M. A. (2020). Strategies to use fibrinogen as bioink for 3D bioprinting fibrin-based soft and hard tissues. *Acta Biomaterialia. 117*, 60-76 https://doi.org/10.1016/j.actbio.2020.09.024.

Dent, E. W., Gupton, S. L., & Gertler, F. B. (2011). The growth cone cytoskeleton in Axon outgrowth and guidance. *Cold Spring Harbor Perspectives in Biology, 3*(3): a001800. https://doi.org/10.1101/cshperspect.a001800.

DePalma, T. J., Sivakumar, H., & Skardal, A. (2022). Strategies for developing complex multi-component in vitro tumor models: Highlights in glioblastoma. *Advanced Drug Delivery Reviews*, *180*, 114067. https://doi.org/10.1016/j.addr.2021.114067.

Dixon, A. R., Jariwala, S. H., Bilis, Z., Loverde, J. R., Pasquina, P. F., & Alvarez, L. M. (2018). Bridging the gap in peripheral nerve repair with 3D printed and bioprinted conduits. *Biomaterials, 186,* 44-63. https://doi.org/10.1016/j.biomaterials.2018.09.010.

Du, X. (2018). Retraction: 3D bio-printing review (IOP Conf. Ser.: Mater. Sci. Eng. 301 012023). *IOP Conference Series: Materials Science and Engineering*. https://doi.org/10.1088/1757-899x/301/1/012169.

Fairbanks, B. D., Schwartz, M. P., Bowman, C. N., Anseth, K. S., Faes, M., Valkenaers, H., Vogeler, F., Vleugels, J., Ferraris, E., Dávila, J. L., d'Ávila, M. A., He, Y., Yang, F., Zhao, H., Gao, Q., Xia, B., Fu, J., Godbout, C., Follonier Castella, L., Heilshorn, S. C. (2019). Assessing bioink shape fidelity to aid material development in 3D bioprinting. *Biofabrication*. 10(1), 014102.

Fantini, V., Bordoni, M., Scocozza, F., Conti, M., Scarian, E., Carelli, S., Di Giulio, A. M., Marconi, S., Pansarasa, O., Auricchio, F., & Cereda, C. (2019a). Bioink Composition and Printing Parameters for 3D Modeling Neural Tissue. *Cells, 8*(8), 830. https://doi.org/10.3390/cells8080830.

Fantini, V., Bordoni, M., Scocozza, F., Conti, M., Scarian, E., Carelli, S., Di Giulio, A. M., Marconi, S., Pansarasa, O., Auricchio, F., & Cereda, C. (2019b). Bioink Composition and Printing Parameters for 3D Modeling Neural Tissue. *Cells, 8*(8), 830. https://doi.org/10.3390/cells8080830.

Girão, A. F., Sousa, J., Domínguez-Bajo, A., González-Mayorga, A., Bdikin, I., Pujades-Otero, E., Casañ-Pastor, N., Hortigüela, M. J., Otero-Irurueta, G., Completo, A., Serrano, M. C., & Marques, P. A. A. P. (2020). 3D Reduced Graphene Oxide Scaffolds with a Combinatorial Fibrous-Porous Architecture for Neural Tissue Engineering. *ACS Applied Materials and Interfaces, 12,* 38962–38975. https://doi.org/10.1021/acsami.0c10599.

Gu, B. K., Choi, D. J., Park, S. J., Kim, M. S., Kang, C. M., & Kim, C. H. (2016). 3-dimensional bioprinting for tissue engineering applications. *Biomaterials Research, 20,* 12. https://doi.org/10.1186/s40824-016-0058-2.

Gu, Q., Tomaskovic-Crook, E., Wallace, G. G., & Crook, J. M. (2018). Engineering human neural tissue by 3D bioprinting. *Methods in Molecular Biology, 1758,* 129-138. https://doi.org/10.1007/978-1-4939-7741-3_10.

Guillot, A., Collet, C., Nguyen, V. A., Malouin, F., Richards, C., & Doyon, J. (2008). Functional neuroanatomical networks associated with expertise in motor imagery. *NeuroImage, 41*(4), 1471-83. https://doi.org/10.1016/j.neuroimage.2008.03.042.

Haring, A. P., Sontheimer, H., & Johnson, B. N. (2017). Microphysiological human brain and neural systems-on-a-chip: potential alternatives to small animal models and emerging platforms for drug discovery and personalized medicine. *Stem Cell Reviews and Reports*, *13*(3), 381-406 https://doi.org/10.1007/s12015-017-9738-0.

Hendriks, J., Willem Visser, C., Henke, S., Leijten, J., Saris, D. B. F., Sun, C., Lohse, D., & Karperien, M. (2015). Optimizing cell viability in droplet-based cell deposition. *Scientific Reports*, *13*(3), 381-406. https://doi.org/10.1038/srep11304.

Heneka, M. T., Rodríguez, J. J., & Verkhratsky, A. (2010a). Neuroglia in neurodegeneration. *Brain Research Reviews, 63*(1-2), 189-211. https://doi.org/10.1016/j.brainresrev.2009.11.004.

Heneka, M. T., Rodríguez, J. J., & Verkhratsky, A. (2010b). Neuroglia in neurodegeneration. *Brain Research Reviews, 63*(1-2), 189-211. https://doi.org/10.1016/j.brainresrev.2009.11.004.

Hill, P. S. (2009). Regeneration of peripheral nerves using neuroinductive biomaterial scaffolds. *ProQuest Dissertations and Theses*.

Houschyar, K. S., Momeni, A., Pyles, M. N., Cha, J. Y., Maan, Z. N., Duscher, D., Jew, O. S., Siemers, F., & Schoonhoven, J. van. (2016). The role of current techniques and concepts in peripheral nerve repair. *Plastic Surgery International*. https://doi.org/10.1155/2016/4175293.

Hsu, S. H., & Chen, C. W. (2018). 3D bioprinting nerve. *3D Bioprinting for Reconstructive Surgery: Techniques and Applications, 2018,* 355-366. https://doi.org/10.1016/B978-0-08-101103-4.00016-8.

Hubert, C. G., Rivera, M., Spangler, L. C., Wu, Q., Mack, S. C., Prager, B. C., Couce, M., McLendon, R. E., Sloan, A. E., & Rich, J. N. (2016). A three-dimensional organoid culture system derived from human glioblastomas recapitulates the hypoxic gradients and cancer stem cell heterogeneity of tumors found in vivo. *Cancer Research*, *76*(8), 2465–2477. https://doi.org/10.1158/0008-5472.CAN-15-2402.

Iii, V., & Micro, T. (2006). Therapeutic micro/nanotechnology. *BioMEMS and Biomedical Nanotechnology*.

Jacob, F., Salinas, R. D., Zhang, D. Y., Nguyen, P. T. T., Schnoll, J. G., Wong, S. Z. H., Thokala, R., Sheikh, S., Saxena, D., Prokop, S., Liu, D.-A., Qian, X., Petrov, D., Lucas, T., Chen, H. I., Dorsey, J. F., Christian, K. M., Binder, Z. A., Nasrallah, M., Song, H. (2020). A patient-derived glioblastoma organoid model and biobank recapitulates inter- and intra-tumoral heterogeneity. *Cell, 180*(1), 188-204.e22. https://doi.org/10.1016/j.cell.2019.11.036.

Jamieson, C., Keenan, P., Kirkwood, D., Oji, S., Webster, C., Russell, K. A., & Koch, T. G. (2021). A review of recent advances in 3d bioprinting with an eye on future regenerative therapies in veterinary medicine. *Frontiers in Veterinary Science, 7,* 584193. https://doi.org/10.3389/fvets.2020.584193.

Jaqueline L. Vieira, Diego C. Carneiro, Milena B. P. Soares, & Josiane D. V. Barbosa. (2021). Fundamentals of 3D bioprinting technology. *Journal of Bioengineering and Technology Applied to Health, 4*(2), 63-70. https://doi.org/10.34178/jbth.v4i2.162.

Jian, H., Wang, M., Wang, S., Wang, A., & Bai, S. (2018a). 3D bioprinting for cell culture and tissue fabrication. *Bio-Design and Manufacturingi, 1,* 45-61. https://doi.org/10.1007/s42242-018-0006-1.

Jian, H., Wang, M., Wang, S., Wang, A., & Bai, S. (2018b). 3D bioprinting for cell culture and tissue fabrication. *Bio-Design and Manufacturing, 1,* 45-61. https://doi.org/10.1007/s42242-018-0006-1.

Khoshnood, N., & Zamanian, A. (2020). A comprehensive review on scaffold-free bioinks for bioprinting. *Bioprinting, 19,* e00088. https://doi.org/10.1016/j.bprint.2020.e00088.

Kim, J., Ko, I., Seol, Y., Atala, A., Yoo, J. J., & Lee, S. (2016). 3D bioprinting of functional skeletal muscle tissue for volumetric muscle tissue loss. *Tissue Engineering - Part A, 10*(10), 679.

Knowlton, S., Anand, S., Shah, T., & Tasoglu, S. (2018a). Bioprinting for Neural Tissue Engineering. *Trends in Neurosciences, 41*(1), 31-46. https://doi.org/10.1016/j.tins.2017.11.001.

Knowlton, S., Anand, S., Shah, T., & Tasoglu, S. (2018b). Bioprinting for Neural Tissue Engineering. In *Trends in Neurosciences, 41*(1), 31-46. https://doi.org/10.1016/j.tins.2017.11.001.

Knowlton, S., Anand, S., Shah, T., & Tasoglu, S. (2018c). Bioprinting for Neural Tissue Engineering. *Trends in Neurosciences, 41*(1), 31–46. https://doi.org/10.1016/j.tins.2017.11.001.

Koffler, J., Zhu, W., Qu, X., Platoshyn, O., Dulin, J. N., Brock, J., Graham, L., Lu, P., Sakamoto, J., Marsala, M., Chen, S., & Tuszynski, M. H. (2019a). Biomimetic 3D-printed scaffolds for spinal cord injury repair. *Nature Medicine, 25,* 263–269. https://doi.org/10.1038/s41591-018-0296-z.

Koffler, J., Zhu, W., Qu, X., Platoshyn, O., Dulin, J. N., Brock, J., Graham, L., Lu, P., Sakamoto, J., Marsala, M., Chen, S., & Tuszynski, M. H. (2019b). Biomimetic 3D-printed scaffolds for spinal cord injury repair. *Nature Medicine, 25,* 263–269. https://doi.org/10.1038/s41591-018-0296-z.

Kruth, J. P., Leu, M. C., & Nakagawa, T. (1998). Progress in additive manufacturing and rapid prototyping. *CIRP Annals - Manufacturing Technology, 47*(2), 525-540. https://doi.org/10.1016/S0007-8506(07)63240-5.

Lee, C., Abelseth, E., de la Vega, L., & Willerth, S. M. (2019a). Bioprinting a novel glioblastoma tumor model using a fibrin-based bioink for drug screening. *Materials Today Chemistry, 12,* 78-84. https://doi.org/10.1016/j.mtchem.2018.12.005.

Lee, C., Abelseth, E., de la Vega, L., & Willerth, S. M. (2019b). Bioprinting a novel glioblastoma tumor model using a fibrin-based bioink for drug screening. *Materials Today Chemistry, 12,* 78–84. https://doi.org/10.1016/j.mtchem.2018.12.005.

Lee, J., Kotliarova, S., Kotliarov, Y., Li, A., Su, Q., Donin, N. M., Pastorino, S., Purow, B. W., Christopher, N., Zhang, W., Park, J. K., & Fine, H. A. (2006). Tumor stem cells derived from glioblastomas cultured in bFGF and EGF more closely mirror the phenotype and genotype of primary tumors than do serum-cultured cell lines. *Cancer Cell, 9*(5), 391–403. https://doi.org/10.1016/j.ccr.2006.03.030.

Lee, S. J., Esworthy, T., Stake, S., Miao, S., Zuo, Y. Y., Harris, B. T., & Zhang, L. G. (2018a). Advances in 3D Bioprinting for Neural Tissue Engineering. *Advanced Biosystems, 2*(4), 1700213. https://doi.org/10.1002/adbi.201700213.

Lee, S. J., Esworthy, T., Stake, S., Miao, S., Zuo, Y. Y., Harris, B. T., & Zhang, L. G. (2018b). Advances in 3D Bioprinting for Neural Tissue Engineering. *Advanced Biosystems, 2*(4), 1700213. https://doi.org/10.1002/adbi.201700213.

Li, X., Wang, X., Wang, X., Chen, H., Zhang, X., Zhou, L., & Xu, T. (2018). 3D bioprinted rat Schwann cell-laden structures with shape flexibility and enhanced nerve growth factor expression. *3 Biotech 8,* 342. https://doi.org/10.1007/s13205-018-1341-9.

Liao, S. S., Cui, F. Z., Zhang, W., & Feng, Q. L. (2004). Hierarchically biomimetic bone scaffold materials: nano-HA/Collagen/PLA composite. *Journal of Biomedical Materials Research - Part B Applied Biomaterials, 69B*(2), 158-165. https://doi.org/10.1002/jbm.b.20035.

Lindvall, O., & Kokaia, Z. (2006). Stem cells for the treatment of neurological disorders. *Nature. 441*, 1094–1096 https://doi.org/10.1038/nature04960.

Linkous, A., Balamatsias, D., Snuderl, M., Edwards, L., Miyaguchi, K., Milner, T., Reich, B., Cohen-Gould, L., Storaska, A., Nakayama, Y., Schenkein, E., Singhania, R., Cirigliano, S., Magdeldin, T., Lin, Y., Nanjangud, G., Chadalavada, K., Pisapia, D., Liston, C., & Fine, H. A. (2019). Modeling patient-derived glioblastoma with cerebral organoids. *Cell Reports*, *26*(12), 3203-3211.e5. https://doi.org/10.1016/j.celrep.2019.02.063.

Liu, L. J. W., Rosner, J., & Cragg, J. J. (2020). Journal Club: High-dose methylprednisolone for acute traumatic spinal cord injury: A meta-analysis. *Neurology, 95*(6), 272-274. https://doi.org/10.1212/WNL.0000000000009263.

Liu, X., Hao, M., Chen, Z., Zhang, T., Huang, J., Dai, J., & Zhang, Z. (2021a). 3D bio-printed neural tissue constructs for spinal cord injury repair. *Biomaterials, 272,* 120771. https://doi.org/10.1016/j.biomaterials.2021.120771.

Liu, X., Hao, M., Chen, Z., Zhang, T., Huang, J., Dai, J., & Zhang, Z. (2021b). 3D bioprinted neural tissue constructs for spinal cord injury repair. *Biomaterials, 272,* 120771. https://doi.org/10.1016/j.biomaterials.2021.120771.

Liu, Z., Yang, Y., He, L., Pang, M., Luo, C., Liu, B., & Rong, L. (2019). High-dose methylprednisolone for acute traumatic spinal cord injury: A meta-analysis. *Neurology, 93*(9), e841-e850. https://doi.org/10.1212/WNL.0000000000007998.

Logun, M., Zhao, W., Mao, L., & Karumbaiah, L. (2018). Microfluidics in malignant glioma research and precision medicine. *Advanced Biosystems*, *2*(5), 1700221. https://doi.org/10.1002/adbi.201700221.

Lougiaki, P., Tsolaki, M., & Pantazaki, A. (2019). Bioinks and in vitro neurovascular unit production - New prospects in Alzheimer's disease research. *Hellenic Journal of Nuclear Medicine, 22,* 209-222.

Mahumane, G. D., Kumar, P., Du Toit, L. C., Choonara, Y. E., & Pillay, V. (2018). 3D scaffolds for brain tissue regeneration: Architectural challenges. *Biomaterials Science, 6,* 2812-2837. https://doi.org/10.1039/c8bm00422f.

Malda, J., Visser, J., Melchels, F. P., Jüngst, T., Hennink, W. E., Dhert, W. J. A., Groll, J., & Hutmacher, D. W. (2013). 25th anniversary article: Engineering hydrogels for biofabrication. *Advanced Materials, 25*(36), 5011-5028. https://doi.org/10.1002/adma.201302042.

Maloney, E., Clark, C., Sivakumar, H., Yoo, K., Aleman, J., Rajan, S. A. P., Forsythe, S., Mazzocchi, A., Laxton, A. W., Tatter, S. B., Strowd, R. E., Votanopoulos, K. I., & Skardal, A. (2020). Immersion bioprinting of tumor organoids in multi-well plates for increasing chemotherapy screening throughput. *Micromachines, 11*(2), 208. https://doi.org/10.3390/mi11020208.

Matai, I., Kaur, G., Seyedsalehi, A., McClinton, A., & Laurencin, C. T. (2020a). Progress in 3D bioprinting technology for tissue/organ regenerative engineering. *Biomaterials, 226,* 119536. https://doi.org/10.1016/j.biomaterials.2019.119536.

Matai, I., Kaur, G., Seyedsalehi, A., McClinton, A., & Laurencin, C. T. (2020b). Progress in 3D bioprinting technology for tissue/organ regenerative engineering. *Biomaterials, 226,* 119536. https://doi.org/10.1016/j.biomaterials.2019.119536.

Mobaraki, M., Ghaffari, M., Yazdanpanah, A., Luo, Y., & Mills, D. K. (2020a). Bioinks and bioprinting: A focused review. *Bioprinting, 18,* e00080. https://doi.org/10.1016/j.bprint.2020.e00080.

Mobaraki, M., Ghaffari, M., Yazdanpanah, A., Luo, Y., & Mills, D. K. (2020b). Bioinks and bioprinting: A focused review. *Bioprinting, 18,* e00080. https://doi.org/10.1016/j.bprint.2020.e00080.

Ngan, C. G. Y., Quigley, A., Williams, R. J., O'connell, C. D., Blanchard, R., Boyd-Moss, M., Aumann, T. D., McKelvie, P., Wallace, G. G., Choong, P. F. M., & Kapsa, R. M. I. (2021). Matured myofibers in bioprinted constructs with in vivo vascularization and innervation. *Gels, 7*(4), 171. https://doi.org/10.3390/gels7040171.

Ning, L., Sun, H., Lelong, T., Guilloteau, R., Zhu, N., Schreyer, D. J., & Chen, X. (2018a). 3D bioprinting of scaffolds with living Schwann cells for potential nerve tissue engineering applications. *Biofabrication, 10*(3):035014. https://doi.org/10.1088/1758-5090/aacd30.

Ning, L., Sun, H., Lelong, T., Guilloteau, R., Zhu, N., Schreyer, D. J., & Chen, X. (2018b). 3D bioprinting of scaffolds with living Schwann cells for potential nerve tissue engineering applications. *Biofabrication, 10*(3):035014. https://doi.org/10.1088/1758-5090/aacd30.

Ning, L., Zhu, N., Mohabatpour, F., Sarker, M. D., Schreyer, D. J., & Chen, X. (2019). Bioprinting Schwann cell-laden scaffolds from low-viscosity hydrogel compositions. *Journal of Materials Chemistry B, 7,* 4538-4551. https://doi.org/10.1039/c9tb00669a.

Ning, L., Zhu, N., Smith, A., Rajaram, A., Hou, H., Srinivasan, S., Mohabatpour, F., He, L., McLnnes, A., Serpooshan, V., Papagerakis, P., & Chen, X. (2021a). Noninvasive three-dimensional in situ and in vivo characterization of bioprinted hydrogel scaffolds using the x-ray propagation-based imaging technique. *ACS Applied Materials and Interfaces, 13,* 25611–25623. https://doi.org/10.1021/acsami.1c02297.

Ning, L., Zhu, N., Smith, A., Rajaram, A., Hou, H., Srinivasan, S., Mohabatpour, F., He, L., McLnnes, A., Serpooshan, V., Papagerakis, P., & Chen, X. (2021b). Noninvasive three-dimensional in situ and in vivo characterization of bioprinted hydrogel scaffolds using the x-ray propagation-based imaging technique. *ACS Applied Materials and Interfaces, 13,* 25611–25623. https://doi.org/10.1021/acsami.1c02297.

Ogawa, J., Pao, G. M., Shokhirev, M. N., & Verma, I. M. (2018). Glioblastoma model using human cerebral organoids. *Cell Reports*, *23*(4), 1220–1229. https://doi.org/10.1016/j.celrep.2018.03.105.

Oliveira, E. P., Malysz-Cymborska, I., Golubczyk, D., Kalkowski, L., Kwiatkowska, J., Reis, R. L., Oliveira, J. M., & Walczak, P. (2019). Advances in bioinks and in vivo imaging of biomaterials for CNS applications. *Acta Biomaterialia*, *95*, 60-72. https://doi.org/10.1016/j.actbio.2019.05.006.

Orcheston-Findlay, L., Bax, S., Utama, R., Engel, M., Govender, D., & O'neill, G. (2021). Advanced spheroid, tumouroid and 3d bioprinted in-vitro models of adult and paediatric glioblastoma. *International Journal of Molecular Sciences*, *22*(6), 1–19. https://doi.org/10.3390/ijms22062962.

Owens, C., Marga, F., & Forgacs, G. (2015a). Bioprinting of nerve. *Essentials of 3D Biofabrication and Translation, 2015*, 379-394. https://doi.org/10.1016/B978-0-12-800972-7.00023-2.

Owens, C., Marga, F., & Forgacs, G. (2015b). Chapter 23 – Bioprinting of Nerve. *Essentials of 3D Biofabrication and Translation, 2015*, 379-394.

Ozbolat, I. T., & Hospodiuk, M. (2016). Current advances and future perspectives in extrusion-based bioprinting. *Biomaterials*. https://doi.org/10.1016/j.biomaterials.2015.10.076.

Panigada, M., Mietto, C., Pagan, F., Bogno, L., Berto, V., & Gattinoni, L. (2013). Monitoring anticoagulation during extracorporeal membrane oxygenation in patients with acute respiratory failure. *Critical Care, 76,* 321-343. https://doi.org/10.1186/cc12064.

Peng, W., Datta, P., Ayan, B., Ozbolat, V., Sosnoski, D., & Ozbolat, I. T. (2017). 3D bioprinting for drug discovery and development in pharmaceutics. *Acta Biomaterialia, 57,* 26-46. https://doi.org/10.1016/j.actbio.2017.05.025.

Petcu, E. B., Midha, R., McColl, E., Popa-Wagner, A., Chirila, T. V., & Dalton, P. D. (2018). 3D printing strategies for peripheral nerve regeneration. *Biofabrication, 10*(3). https://doi.org/10.1088/1758-5090/aaaf50.

Pollard, K. J., Sharma, A. D., & Moore, M. J. (2019). Neural microphysiological systems for in vitro modeling of peripheral nervous system disorders. *Bioelectronics in Medicine, 2*(2). https://doi.org/10.2217/bem-2019-0018.

Pollard, S. M., Yoshikawa, K., Clarke, I. D., Danovi, D., Stricker, S., Russell, R., Bayani, J., Head, R., Lee, M., Bernstein, M., Squire, J. A., Smith, A., & Dirks, P. (2009). Glioma stem cell lines expanded in adherent culture have tumor-specific phenotypes and are suitable for chemical and genetic screens. *Cell Stem Cell*, *4*(6), 568–580. https://doi.org/10.1016/j.stem.2009.03.014.

Pontén, J., & Macintyre, E. H. (1968). Long term culture of normal and neoplastic human glia. *Acta Pathologica et Microbiologica Scandinavica*, *74*(4), 465–486. https://doi.org/10.1111/j.1699-0463.1968.tb03502.x.

Purves, D., Augustine, G. J., Fitzpatrick, D., Hall, W. C., Lamantia, A.-S., & White, L. E. (2013). Neuroscienze. *Neuroscience*, Oxford University Press.

Qian, T., Guo, X., Levi, A. D., Vanni, S., Shebert, R. T., & Sipski, M. L. (2005). High-dose methylprednisolone may cause myopathy in acute spinal cord injury patients. *Spinal Cord, 43,* 199–203. https://doi.org/10.1038/sj.sc.3101681.

Restan Perez, M., Sharma, R., Masri, N. Z., & Willerth, S. M. (2021). 3D bioprinting mesenchymal stem cell-derived neural tissues using a fibrin-based bioink. *Biomolecules, 11(8),* 1250. https://doi.org/10.3390/biom11081250.

Rivetti di Val Cervo, P., Besusso, D., Conforti, P., & Cattaneo, E. (2021). hiPSCs for predictive modelling of neurodegenerative diseases: dreaming the possible. *Nature Reviews Neurology*, *17*(6), 381–392. https://doi.org/10.1038/s41582-021-00465-0.

Rothenbücher, T. S. P., & Martínez-Serrano, A. (2019). Human cerebral organoids and neural 3D tissues in basic research, and their application to study neurological diseases. *Future Neurology, 14*(1). https://doi.org/10.2217/fnl-2018-0043.

Rybin, M. J., Ivan, M. E., Ayad, N. G., & Zeier, Z. (2021). Organoid models of glioblastoma and their role in drug discovery. *Frontiers in Cellular Neuroscience, 15*(February), 1–11. https://doi.org/10.3389/fncel.2021.605255.

Sahai, N., & Gogoi, M. (2019). Techniques and software used in 3D printing for nanomedicine applications. *3D Printing Technology in Nanomedicine, 2019,* 23-41. https://doi.org/10.1016/B978-0-12-815890-6.00002-5.

Saliba, J., Daou, A., Damiati, S., Saliba, J., El-Sabban, M., & Mhanna, R. (2018a). Development of microplatforms to mimic the in vivo architecture of CNS and PNS physiology and their diseases. *Genes, 9*(6), 285. https://doi.org/10.3390/genes 9060285.

Saliba, J., Daou, A., Damiati, S., Saliba, J., El-Sabban, M., & Mhanna, R. (2018b). Development of microplatforms to mimic the in vivo architecture of CNS and PNS physiology and their diseases. *Genes, 9*(6), 285. https://doi.org/10.3390/genes9060285.

Salles, G. N., Calió, M. L., Holscher, C., Pacheco-Soares, C., Porcionatto, M., & Oliveira Lobo, A. (2018). P3-067: Poly(Lactic Acid) (Pla) Electrospun fibers improve neurogenesis and reduce β-amyloid plaques in a transgenic mouse model of alzheimer's disease. *Alzheimer's & Dementia, 14*(75), 1090. https://doi.org/10.1016/j.jalz.2018.06.1423.

Sarker, M. D., Naghieh, S., McInnes, A. D., Schreyer, D. J., & Chen, X. (2018). Regeneration of peripheral nerves by nerve guidance conduits: Influence of design, biopolymers, cells, growth factors, and physical stimuli. *Progress in Neurobiology, 171,* 125-150. https://doi.org/10.1016/j.pneurobio.2018.07.002.

Sekhon, L. H. S., & Fehlings, M. G. (2001). Epidemiology, demographics, and pathophysiology of acute spinal cord injury. *Spine, 26*(24S), S2-S12. https://doi.org/10.1097/00007632-200112151-00002.

Sharma, R., Smits, I. P. M., De La Vega, L., Lee, C., & Willerth, S. M. (2020a). 3D bioprinting pluripotent stem cell derived neural tissues using a novel fibrin bioink containing drug releasing microspheres. *Frontiers in Bioengineering and Biotechnology, 8, 57*. https://doi.org/10.3389/fbioe.2020.00057.

Sharma, R., Smits, I. P. M., De La Vega, L., Lee, C., & Willerth, S. M. (2020b). 3D Bioprinting pluripotent stem cell derived neural tissues using a novel fibrin bioink containing drug releasing microspheres. *Frontiers in Bioengineering and Biotechnology, 8, 57*. https://doi.org/10.3389/fbioe.2020.00057.

Shiju, T. M., Carlos de Oliveira, R., & Wilson, S. E. (2020). 3D in vitro corneal models: A review of current technologies. *Experimental Eye Research, 200,* 108213. https://doi.org/10.1016/j.exer.2020.108213.

Silvani, G., Basirun, C., Wu, H., Mehner, C., Poole, K., Bradbury, P., & Chou, J. (2021). A 3D-bioprinted vascularized glioblastoma-on-a-chip for studying the impact of simulated microgravity as a novel pre-clinical approach in brain tumor therapy. *Advanced Therapeutics*, *4*(11), 1–14. https://doi.org/10.1002/adtp.202100106.

Slanzi, A., Iannoto, G., Rossi, B., Zenaro, E., & Constantin, G. (2020). In vitro models of neurodegenerative diseases. *Frontiers in Cell and Developmental Biology*, *8*, 328. https://doi.org/10.3389/fcell.2020.00328.

Soman, P., Tobe, B. T. D., Lee, J. W., Winquist, A. M., Singec, I., Vecchio, K. S., Snyder, E. Y., & Chen, S. (2012). Three-dimensional scaffolding to investigate neuronal derivatives of human embryonic stem cells. *Biomedical Microdevices, 14,* 829-838. https://doi.org/10.1007/s10544-012-9662-7.

Song, D., Xu, Y., Liu, S., Wen, L., & Wang, X. (2021). Progress of 3d bioprinting in organ manufacturing. *Polymers, 13*(18), 3178. https://doi.org/10.3390/polym13183178.

Song, S., Liu, X., Huang, J., & Zhang, Z. (2022). Neural stem cell-laden 3D bioprinting of polyphenol-doped electroconductive hydrogel scaffolds for enhanced neuronal differentiation. *Materials Science and Engineering: C*, 112639. https://doi.org/10.1016/j.msec.2021.112639.

Stapenhorst, F., Garrido dos Santos, M., Prestes, J. P., Alcantara, B. J., Felisberto Borges, M., & Pranke, P. (2021). Bioprinting: A promising approach for tissue regeneration. *Bioprinting, 22,* e00130. https://doi.org/10.1016/j.bprint.2021.e00130.

Subramanian, A., Krishnan, U. M., & Sethuraman, S. (2009a). Development of biomaterial scaffold for nerve tissue engineering: Biomaterial mediated neural regeneration. *Journal of Biomedical Science*, *108*(2009). https://doi.org/10.1186/1423-0127-16-108.

Subramanian, A., Krishnan, U. M., & Sethuraman, S. (2009b). Development of biomaterial scaffold for nerve tissue engineering: Biomaterial mediated neural regeneration. *Journal of Biomedical Science*, *108*(2009). https://doi.org/10.1186/1423-0127-16-108.

Subramanian, A., Krishnan, U. M., & Sethuraman, S. (2011). Skin tissue regeneration. In *Electrospinning for Tissue Regeneration*, 298-316. https://doi.org/10.1016/B978-1-84569-741-9.50014-8.

Tan, S. K., Jermakowicz, A., Mookhtiar, A. K., Nemeroff, C. B., Schürer, S. C., & Ayad, N. G. (2018). Drug repositioning in glioblastoma: A pathway perspective. *Frontiers in Pharmacology*, *9*(MAR), 218. https://doi.org/10.3389/fphar.2018.00218.

Tang, M., Tiwari, S. K., Agrawal, K., Tan, M., Dang, J., Tam, T., Tian, J., Wan, X., Schimelman, J., You, S., Xia, Q., Rana, T. M., & Chen, S. (2021). Rapid 3D bioprinting of glioblastoma model mimicking native biophysical heterogeneity. *Small*, *17*(15), 1–13. https://doi.org/10.1002/smll.202006050.

Thakkar, J. P., Dolecek, T. A., Horbinski, C., Ostrom, Q. T., Lightner, D. D., Barnholtz-Sloan, J. S., & Villano, J. L. (2014). Epidemiologic and molecular prognostic review of glioblastoma. *Cancer Epidemiology Biomarkers and Prevention*, *23*(10), 1985–1996. https://doi.org/10.1158/1055-9965.EPI-14-0275.

Tian, T., & Li, X. (2020). Applications of tissue clearing in the spinal cord. In *European Journal of Neuroscience, 52*(9), 4019-4036. https://doi.org/10.1111/ejn.14938.

Tortorella, S., Greco, P., Valle, F., Barbalinardo, M., Foschi, G., Lugli, F., Dallavalle, M., Zerbetto, F., Bortolotti, C. A., & Biscarini, F. (2022). Laser Assisted Bioprinting of laminin on biodegradable PLGA substrates: Effect on neural stem cell adhesion and differentiation. *Bioprinting*, e00194. https://doi.org/https://doi.org/10.1016/j.bprint.2022.e00194.

Uemura, T., Takamatsu, K., Ikeda, M., Okada, M., Kazuki, K., Ikada, Y., & Nakamura, H. (2011). A tissue-engineered bioabsorbable nerve conduit created by three-dimensional culture of induced pluripotent stem cell-derived neurospheres. *Bio-Medical Materials and Engineering, 2011,* 331-339. https://doi.org/10.3233/BME-2012-0680.

Venugopal, C., Chandanala, S., Prasad, H. C., Nayeem, D., Bhonde, R. R., & Dhanushkodi, A. (2017). Regenerative therapy for hippocampal degenerative diseases: lessons from preclinical studies. *Journal of Tissue Engineering and Regenerative Medicine, 11*(2), 321-333. https://doi.org/10.1002/term.2052.

Wang, X., He, J., Wang, Y., & Cui, F. Z. (2012). Hyaluronic acid-based scaffold for central neural tissue engineering. *Interface Focus*. https://doi.org/10.1098/rsfs.2012.0016.

Wang, X., Li, X., Ding, J., Long, X., Zhang, H., Zhang, X., Jiang, X., & Xu, T. (2021). 3D bioprinted glioma microenvironment for glioma vascularization. *Journal of Biomedical Materials Research - Part A, 109*(6), 915–925. https://doi.org/10.1002/jbm.a.37082.

Wang, X., Yan, Y., & Zhang, R. (2007). Rapid prototyping as a tool for manufacturing bioartificial livers. *Trends in Biotechnology, 25*(11), 505-513. https://doi.org/10.1016/j.tibtech.2007.08.010.

Wang, Y., Li, J., Li, Y., & Yang, B. (2021a). Biomimetic bioinks of nanofibrillar polymeric hydrogels for 3D bioprinting. *Nano Today, 39*(2021), 101180. https://doi.org/10.1016/j.nantod.2021.101180.

Wang, Y., Li, J., Li, Y., & Yang, B. (2021b). Biomimetic bioinks of nanofibrillar polymeric hydrogels for 3D bioprinting. *Nano Today, 39*(2021), 101180. https://doi.org/10.1016/j.nantod.2021.101180.

Wang, Z., Kapadia, W., Li, C., Lin, F., Pereira, R. F., Granja, P. L., Sarmento, B., & Cui, W. (2021). Tissue-specific engineering: 3D bioprinting in regenerative medicine. In *Journal of Controlled Release, 329,* 237-256. https://doi.org/10.1016/j.jconrel.2020.11.044.

Witthayanuwat, S., Pesee, M., Supaadirek, C., Supakalin, N., Thamronganantasakul, K., & Krusun, S. (2018). Survival analysis of Glioblastoma Multiforme. *Asian Pacific Journal of Cancer Prevention, 19*(9), 2613–2617. https://doi.org/10.22034/APJCP.2018.19.9.2613.

Wong, K. V., & Hernandez, A. (2012). A review of additive manufacturing. *ISRN Mechanical Engineering, 2012,* 1-10. https://doi.org/10.5402/2012/208760.

Xue, W., Shi, W., Kong, Y., Kuss, M., & Duan, B. (2021). Anisotropic scaffolds for peripheral nerve and spinal cord regeneration. *Bioactive Materials, 6*(11), 4141-4160. https://doi.org/10.1016/j.bioactmat.2021.04.019.

Yi, H. G., Jeong, Y. H., Kim, Y., Choi, Y. J., Moon, H. E., Park, S. H., Kang, K. S., Bae, M., Jang, J., Youn, H., Paek, S. H., & Cho, D.-W. (2019). A bioprinted human-glioblastoma-on-a-chip for the identification of patient-specific responses to chemoradiotherapy. *Nature Biomedical Engineering*, *3*(7), 509–519. https://doi.org/10.1038/s41551-019-0363-x.

Yilmaz, B., Tahmasebifar, A., & Baran, E. T. (2020). Bioprinting technologies in tissue engineering. In *Advances in Biochemical Engineering/Biotechnology,* 279-319. https://doi.org/10.1007/10_2019_108.

Yoo, J., Wilson, W. C., Boland, T., Xu, T., Willeme, F., Wikipedia, Wan, X., Li, D., Zhang, S., Ussyshkin, V., Theriault, L., The Complete University Guide, TFE COATING, Tesla, N., Terrell, D. L., Tan, Y., Zhu, K., Zhang, S., Strategyzer. 3 dynamics system. (2017a). *Bioscaffolder 3.1*. Biofabrication.

Yoo, J., Wilson, W. C., Boland, T., Xu, T., Willeme, F., Wikipedia, Wan, X., Li, D., Zhang, S., Ussyshkin, V., Theriault, L., The Complete University Guide, TFE COATING, Tesla, N., Terrell, D. L., Tan, Y., Zhu, K., Zhang, S., Strategyzer. 3 Dynamics System. (2017b). *Bioscaffolder 3.1*. Biofabrication.

Yu, X., Zhang, T., & Li, Y. (2020). 3D printing and bioprinting nerve conduits for neural tissue engineering. *Polymers, 12*(8), 1637. https://doi.org/10.3390/POLYM12081637.

Zhang, L. G., & Kaplan, D. L. (2016). Neural engineering: From advanced biomaterials to 3D fabrication techniques. *Neural Engineering: From Advanced Biomaterials to 3D Fabrication Techniques,* Springer. https://doi.org/10.1007/978-3-319-31433-4.

Zhang, L., Wang, J. J. J. C. J., Feng, X., Cai, W., Yang, J., Zhang, N., Bue, M., Hanberg, P., Tøttrup, M., Thomassen, M. B., Birke-Sørensen, H., Thillemann, T. M., Andersson, T. L., Søballe, K., Shiels, S. M., Raut, V. P., Patterson, P. B., Barnes, B. R., Wenke, J. C. Marston, S. B. (2005). Abstracts. *CONNECT: The World of Critical Care Nursing.*

Zhang, Y., Chen, H., Long, X., & Xu, T. (2022). Three-dimensional-engineered bioprinted in vitro human neural stem cell self-assembling culture model constructs of Alzheimer's disease. *Bioactive Materials*, *11*, 192–205. https://doi.org/10.1016/j.bioactmat.2021.09.023.

Zhong, Y., & Bellamkonda, R. V. (2008). Biomaterials for the central nervous system. *Journal of the Royal Society Interface, 5,* 957–975. https://doi.org/10.1098/rsif.2008.0071.

Zhu, W., Castro, N. J., & Zhang, L. G. (2015a). Nanotechnology and 3D Bioprinting for Neural Tissue Regeneration. In *3D Bioprinting and Nanotechnology in Tissue Engineering and Regenerative Medicine, 2015,* 307-331. https://doi.org/10.1016/B978-0-12-800547-7.00014-X.

Zhu, W., Castro, N. J., & Zhang, L. G. (2015b). Nanotechnology and 3D Bioprinting for Neural Tissue Regeneration. In *3D Bioprinting and Nanotechnology in Tissue Engineering and Regenerative Medicine, 2015,* 307-331. https://doi.org/10.1016/B978-0-12-800547-7.00014-X.

Chapter 11

Bioprinting for Solid Organs

Nilsun Kuas*, MD
Department of Pediatric Surgery,
Pediatric Urology, Ankara University,
Ankara, Turkey

Abstract

Transplantation remains the gold standard in the treatment of end-stage organ diseases. However, tissue compatibility is only an option in selected patients for organ transplantation, and the use of continuous immunosuppressive agents is complex (Jorgensen et al., 2020). 3D printing uses computer-controlled systems to create anatomically correct organ biomaterials (with or without cells) to correct geometries. (Schubert et al., 2014). Biomaterials can be used to fabricate organ improvement (Rudolph, 1994). An avascular network is essential to combine and deliver nutrients and oxygen (Jia et al., 2016). Organ-specific microstructures are essential for the proper functioning of all bioprinted organs. They consist of a complex fashion with complex and delicate structural elements composed of multiple cell types (Jorgensen et al., 2020).

Keywords: bioprinting, organs, bioengineering

* Corresponding Author's Email: dr.nilsun@hotmail.com.

In: Bioprinting the Human
Editors: Soner Şahin and Kenan Demir
ISBN: 978-1-68507-993-2

Introduction

The field of tissue engineering is heading toward total organ transplantation (Jorgensen et al., 2020). Tissue engineering emphasizes the renewal of solitary tissues and organs based on medical progress, allowing scientists to reconstruct compound tissues (Abdollahiyan et al., 2021). Nanotechnology has appeared to be a brilliant way to guide issues toward programmed differentiation (Dang et al., 2018; Fahy et al., 2018).

Organ transplantation only in selected patients, the search for tissue compatibility, and the continuous use of immunosuppressive agents limit treatment. So, the priority target of bioengineers is to produce solid organs from patient-specific cells. Engineered tubular, hollow, and flat organs have already been successfully created and transplanted. Nevertheless, this has not yet been successful for solid organs.

Today's best way to engineer solid organs is through 3D bioprinting (Jorgensen et al., 2020). 3D printing uses computer-controlled systems to create anatomically correct organs. Biomaterials (with or without cells) are used to correct geometries (Schubert et al., 2014). Cells can be isolated from patients to expand and enable autologous implants (Albanna et al., 2019). Finally, biomaterials can be used to fabricate organ improvement (Rudolph, 1994). For all of this, correct biomaterial plans are essential for direct cell self-assembly (Stupp, 2010). Macrostructural organ involutions include flat tissue, tubular structures, hollow structures, and solid organs. Because all organs must have adult vascular networks to survive, solid organs are the most complex. In addition, organs have multiple cell types, which requires a more complex organization (Jorgensen et al., 2020). An avascular network will be critical to combine and deliver nutrients and oxygen (Jia et al., 2016).

To replicate the properties of the extracellular matrix, tunable biomaterials are used. These are naturally produced materials used for organ bioprinting. They are designed to promote self-assembly into microstructures and proliferation (Jorgensen et al., 2020). These substrates describe tissue construction plans (Das et al., 2015). Appropriate physiological conditions must exist in cell-laden scaffolds, such as desired nutrients and oxygen levels (Abdollahiyan et al., 2021). In theory, a scaffold should be a quick process that degrades and reabsorbs over time (Stupp, 2010). Tissue engineering techniques are efficient simply by the biologically activated factor of cells (Peneda Pacheco et al., 2021; Zhang et al., 2009). There are two types of scaffolds; biomaterial-based and acellular-based scaffolds (Abdollahiyan et al., 2021).

In the last decade, collagen-based biomaterials have been widely used because collagen is the most common protein in the human body that can be extracted, polymerized and proliferated (Cui et al., 2017; Jorgensen et al., 2020). In addition, other biomaterials such as alginate, fibrinogen, gelatin, hyaluronic acid, agarose, and silk (Jorgensen et al., 2020). In addition, nural polymers may not be precisely expected or controllable because of their degradation rate (Neubauer et al., 2021).

There are also synthetic polymers such as polyethylene glycol (PEG) and polyurethane. These are flexible for chemical modification (Jorgensen et al., 2020). The hydrolytic degradation behavior is the critical point and is more predictable and controllable than enzymatic polymers (Abdollahiyan et al., 2021). Because of the acidic nature of the atrophied remnants, some materials may trigger a prolonged inflammatory response (Salazar-Noratto et al., 2020). Polymeric biomaterials provide greater control over the physicochemical properties of scaffolds (Abdollahiyan et al., 2021).

Most methods must work with biomaterials, but other methods require media-based liquid cell suspensions, including inkjet bioprinting (Jorgensen et al., 2020). Media-based printing is balanced on media and meticulously extruded to spesific locations (Phillippi et al., 2008). This method has been used to fabricate kidney microstructures (Faulkner-Jones et al., 2013). In another method of using media for bioprinting has cell spheroids are inflated into a needle assembly. The spheroids are then self-assembled to form solid tissues (Jorgensen et al., 2020). This scaffold-free approach has formed liver microstructures and cardiac patches (Kizawa et al., 2017; Ong et al., 2017). In addition, Nakayama et al. recorded that human embryonic stem cells diffrentiated into kidney-like cells after impregnation with monkey kidney decellularized scaffolds. However, this was not monitored in acellular lung tissues (LoPresti & Brown, 2018).

The configuration of the vascular tissue includes three layers of extracellular matrix and cells (Stegemann et al., 2007). A maximum distance of 300μm seperates arterioles. Besides, the vascular formation can control tissue formation itself (Rouwkema et al., 2008; Zhang et al., 2009). Therefore, the first effort to replicate vascular tissue includes manufactured vascular grafts.

Nevertheless, these were effective only in large (> 8mm) and medium-sized vessels. To stimulate infiltration of blood vessels, growth factors are used or a technique called indirect printing is employed. In addition, luminal support made of sacrificial materials can maintain an open internal lumen during vessel formation (Jorgensen et al., 2020).

Solid Organs

Organ-specific microstructures are critical for the proper functioning of all bioprinted organ complexes, and delicate structural elements are composed of multiple cell types.

Hepatic tissue consists of hepatocytes, Kupffer cells, stromal cells, and cells associated with blood vessels, which are organized cells tunneled through bile ducts and blood vessels (Jorgensen et al., 2020). For culture, primary hepatocytes could not survive for an extended period of time, so a synthetic liver was also thwarted (Y. Kim et al., 2017). Hepatocytes have a high proliferative capacity in vivo and represent 60% of the liver volume. However, in in vitro culture, cells can lose their specific function (Jorgensen et al., 2020). Unexpectedly, organ function requires 30%, but this is still a challenge (Brovold et al., 2018). Autologous liver stem cells are the first choice as a cell source, but, like iPSCs, mesenchymal SCs and humanized hepatocytes are also alternatives. (Agmon & Christman, 2016; Kadota et al., 2014). Researchers have decellularized the liver ECM in different ways (Jaramillo et al., 2018; Kakabadze et al., 2018). First, decellularization is obtained by pumping detergents through the portal vein with peristaltic pumps. Then Baptista and colleagues tried to reintroduce cells into the decellularized scaffold (Baptista et al., 2011, 2013). Reendothelization of vascular tissue was improved by the use of anti-VD31 antibodies by Ko et al., in 2015 (Ko et al., 2015b).

In their study of liver production, Bhatia et al., announced that they had produced organized tissue units human hepatocytes and fibroblasts with endothelial cords (Stevens et al., 2017b). After implantation into a mouse, the tissues grew 50-fold and produced multiple liver proteins (Jorgensen et al., 2020). Other studies used a three-dimensional synthetic scaffold of biodelactic polylactic acid seeded with hepatocytes to improve cellular transplantation (Y. Kim et al., 2017). Endothelial cells and hepatocytes were produced as monolayers. Eventually, both cell forms were preserved and albumin production was maintained by hepatocytes (Jorgensen et al., 2020). Later research showed that photocrosslinkable polyethylene glycol (PEG) could maintain hepatocellular function in bioprintable hydrogels. (Underhill et al., 2007). Bhatia et al., produced a photopatterning platform using liver tissue, then used to embed cells in hydrogels with multiple layers (Tsang et al., 2007). Transplantation of human ectopic artificial livers (HEALs) into mice exhibited human liver functions, such as human drug metabolism and human protein synthesis (Chen et al., 2011). The group also used inVERT molding (Intaglio-Void/Embed-Relief Topographic molding). Thus, liver functions were modulated, including compartment microstructure and microscale induced pluripotent stem cells (Stevens et al., 2013). Later, primary rat hepatocytes were printed using an extrusion bioprinter. In the project, the skeleton was formed with polycaprolactone. Then the collagen bioink and cells were infused into the auxiliary structure. The 3D coculture atmosphere stimulated capillary production, and facilitated growth of the liver cells (Jorgensen et al., 2020).

The respiratory system extracts oxygen from the atmosphere and removes gaseous waste from the body. The epithelial cells of the respiratory system are located between the outer atmosphere and the internal organs. This tissue is a barrier against inhaled irritants; it must also cooperate with the immune system (Brovold et al., 2018). Investigators have made several attempts to produce lung tissue, but the 3D alveolar model has not yet been functionally built (Jaramillo et al., 2018; Kakabadze et al., 2018). Alveolar sacs are 200 micrometers in diameter and have a complex branched network of capillaries and airway membranes.

Mockros et al., planned the technique of performing up to hundreds of millions of parallel lithographs to create three-dimensional arrays of gas pathways and blood microchannels in PDMS (polydimethylsiloxane) to test gas permeability. They have reduced the risk of thrombosis by lining the capillary network with endothelial cells. The same technology was used to develop a lung assist device for patients suffering from failing lungs and awaiting transplantation (Jorgensen et al., 2020). Klein et al., produced a system in which different cells were implanted onto a microporous membrane to pretend the alveolar surface. The system thus created allowed us to study the toxic effects of granules (Klein et al., 2013).

Hug et al., designed a human cell-based lung on a chip. They designed an alveolar-capillary barrier in a thin PDMS membrane covered with ECM, mimicking physiological respiratory activities (Huh et al., 2010). This study mimics the microarchitecture of the alveolar capillary unit and can be used for drug studies (Brovold et al., 2018). Following the decellularization approach, several other groups have studied cell seeding, a technique to protect the compound microstructural netting of human lung tissues. Researchers examined whether lung tissue can be restored in vitro. They preserved components of the extracellular matrix while removing the cellular parts of the rat lung. The components of the decellularized extracellular matrix were seeded with vascular endothelium and lung epithelium in a bioreactor. They found that the endothelium mimicked the vasculature. When transplanted into rats, artificial alveolar tissues participated in gas exchange (Jorgensen et al.,

2020). These results suggest that seeding cells in the ECM is likely to produce lung tissue (Pagliuca et al., 2014).

Panoskaltsis Mortari developed a lung matrix bioreactor to reproduce decellularized tissue by perfusion of detergent implanted in cells. The mouse lung matrix was first decellularized and then transferred to a ventilator. The matrix did not deteriorate over time as it pretended to breathe. Instead, the researchers designed a microphysiological organoid with a functional alveolar- alveolar-capillary interface like the human lung. When inflammatory cytokines and bacteria were introduced into the alveolar area produced in the rat body, the system triggered a biomimetic response. (Jorgensen et al., 2020).

The kidney is one of the most complicated organ due to its particular development with intricately patterned epithelial tubes, the nephrons, and 30 different cell types (Baptista et al., 2013). As a result, conventional tissue engineering methods cannot be reproduced in the kidneys (Jorgensen et al., 2020). However, some research institutes have attempted to use acellular ECM plans (Kim et al., 1998; Stevens et al., 2013b). These fabricated tissues mimic plasma filtration into a urine-like extract. However, they cannot perform other kidney functions, such as control of vascular blood pressure (Underhill et al., 2007).

Little et al., identified the developmental steps of the progenitor cells that make up the kidney mesenchyme and the collecting duct, corresponding to the development of human kidneys in the first trimester. These descriptions were used to fabricate kidney organoids that contain an organized collecting duct network, including endothelial cells and the renal interstitium (Jorgensen et al., 2020). These fabricated kidney organoids can be used in future disease modeling studies and nephrotoxicity.

Abolbashari et al., used adult renal cells separated from the different cortical segments of the kidney. In addition, the cells expressed other proteins from the proximal tubular cells. The cells expressed other proteins from proximal tubular cells. When the proteins were seeded in scaffolds, they showed good electrolyte absorption, erythropoietin production, and hydrolase activity (Baptista et al., 2013).

Stem cell-based methods are evolving to enable more complex methods of kidney engineering (Jorgensen et al., 2020). Replicating primary developmental marks in vitro can allow human pluripotent stem cells to differentiate into renal cell types such as tubular cells and podocytes, which are typically lost in renal diseases (Baptista et al., 2013). iPSC-derived podocytes are functionally and morphologically similar to human kidney podocyte cells, including the location of the podocyte marker nephrin, Wilm's tumor protein, synaptopodin, and can develop into glomeruli tissues (Jorgensen et al., 2020). Technology can improve the use of tissue spheroids, chip platforms, and the development of the technique to generate glomerulus-specific cells and translate them into more hybrid approaches (Baptista et al., 2013). To test this combination technique, differentiated hiPS cells, reproduced podocytes, and human glomerular endothelial cells were co-cultured in a microfluidic device. The cells formed a biomimetic glomerulus that can induce the clearance of insulin and albumin (Jorgensen et al., 2020). The researchers used cells from a patient with congenital nephrotic syndrome that grew into a glomerular organoid. The organoid had reduced levels of nephrin and podocin protein (Ko et al., 2015b).

Lewis et al., have additionally matured complex three-dimensional kidney tissue models printed on an extracellular matrix with convoluted complex open lumen structures. First, the tube was seeded with epithelial cells from the proximal tubule, improving epithelial functionality and morphology. The researchers then added tubules with confluent epithelium and endothelium with unassisted closed-loop perfusion. This system can exchange solutes, albumin uptake, and glucose reabsorption (Jorgensen et al., 2020). Then, when generated with hyperglycemia, it creates a diseased human-like condition that can be saved by implementing a glucose transport inhibitor (Ko et al., 2015).

Cho et al., have used coaxial printing and functional hybrid bioink to develop recessed microfluidic tubes with renal parenchyma derived from endothelial cells and renal tubule epithelium (Stevens et al., 2017b). By selecting bioactive biomaterials and fabricating the renal tubules, functional kidney units on a chip and implantable constructs can be produced.

The next step in the developing of a functional nephron may be the isolation of specific proximal tubule cells or the differentiation of these cells from progenitor precursors (Jorgensen et al., 2020). In addition, renal organoids can provide information about nephrogenesis and are useful development accuracy (Little & Combes, 2019).

Scaffolds can be made to mimic the microenvironment of the pancreas. The surface and porous channels can induce blood vessels to increase oxygen and nutrient uptake (Ko et al., 2015). ECM proteins are deposited in biodegradable scaffold tissue surrounding the scaffolds and then progressively colonized with islets (Stevens et al., 2017). The researchers focused on finding an optimal site for islet transplantation, which was then transplanted into the epididymal fat pad of diabetic rats. The omental pouch has also been studied as an alternative place. The transplanted rats became normoglycemic. However, the scaffolds made progress faster and less than 45% of the rats were kept alive (Jorgensen et al., 2020). The results demonstrate that the scaffolds were efficient for islet transplantation (S. S. Kim et al., 1998). Transplantation was delayed in omental sac recipients, but protein production was similar, making them an alternative (Berman et al., 2009).

All extrahepatic islet cell transplants need stable porous structures for vascularization. Bioprinting was used to produce a 3D alginate-based porous scaffold to improve the surface area for increased nutrient and oxygen transport needs. Although the method prevented cell aggregation, the viability and morphology of β-cell islands did not change during embedding function (Jorgensen et al., 2020). After transplantation to rats, they have maintained their structural integrity and improved cell function (Stevens et al., 2017).

Shea et al., have fabricated a scaffold with microporous biomaterials to guide pancreatic progenitor cells. This scaffold allowed differentiation of the accumulation of pancreatic progenitor cells into clusters. In addition, insulin expression and secretion in response to glucose increased according to culture in suspension (Kim et al., 1998).

Conclusion

3D bioprinting has reformed the field of organ engineering (Stevens et al., 2017). Despite significant advances in tissue engineering, the bioprinting of solid organs has not yet made it possible to transplant diseased organs with fabricated ones. However, engineers have made significant progress thanks to the complete vascularization of decellularized organs and prevention of thrombosis. Autologous iPSCs can be used as a leading cellular resource for recellularized organ tissues (Brovold et al., 2018).

Implementation techniques and technologies have demonstrated that the 3D macrostructure of organs can be fabricated functionally. In addition, further advances in the field have enabled the fabrication of small-diameter blood vessels to enable organ engineering with perfusion. Finally, biomaterials development has led to tunable bioinks that reproduce nanostructural organ tissues such as the ECM, which are necessary to support cellular expansion and replication (Jorgensen et al., 2020).

References

Abdollahiyan, P., Oroojalian, F., Hejazi, M., de la Guardia, M., & Mokhtarzadeh, A. (2021). Nanotechnology, and scaffold implantation for the effective repair of injured organs: An overview on hard tissue engineering. *Journal of Controlled Release*, *333*, 391–417. https://doi.org/10.1016/j.jconrel.2021.04.003.

Agmon, G., & Christman, K. L. (2016). Controlling stem cell behavior with decellularized extracellular matrix scaffolds. *Current Opinion in Solid State and Materials Science*, *20*(4), 193–201. https://doi.org/10.1016/j.cossms.2016.02.001.

Albanna, M., Binder, K. W., Murphy, S. v., Kim, J., Qasem, S. A., Zhao, W., Tan, J., El-Amin, I. B., Dice, D. D., Marco, J., Green, J., Xu, T., Skardal, A., Holmes, J. H., Jackson, J. D., Atala, A., & Yoo, J. J. (2019). In situ bioprinting of autologous skin cells accelerates wound healing of extensive excisional full-thickness wounds. *Scientific Reports*, *9*(1), 1–15. https://doi.org/10.1038/s41598-018-38366-w.

Baptista, P.M., Siddiqui, M. M., Lozier, G., Rodriguez, S. R., Atala, A., & Soker, S. (2011). The use of whole organ decellularization for the generation of a vascularized liver organoid. *Hepatology*, *53*(2), 604–617. https://doi.org/10.1002/hep.24067.

Baptista, P.M., Vyas, D., Moran, E., Wang, Z., & Soker, S. (2013). Human liver bioengineering using a whole liver decellularized bioscaffold. *Methods in Molecular Biology*, *1001*, 289–298. https://doi.org/10.1007/978-1-62703-363-3_24.

Berman, D. M., O'Neil, J. J., Coffey, L. C. K., Chaffanjon, P. C. J., Kenyon, N. M., Ruiz, P., Pileggi, A., Ricordi, C., & Kenyon, N. S. (2009). Long-term survival of nonhuman primate islets implanted in an omental pouch on a biodegradable scaffold. *American Journal of Transplantation*, *9*(1), 91–104. https://doi.org/10.1111/j.1600-6143.2008.02489.x.

Brovold, M., Almeida, J. I., Pla-Palacín, I., Sainz-Arnal, P., Sánchez-Romero, N., Rivas, J. J., Almeida, H., Dachary, P. R., Serrano-Aulló, T., Soker, S., & Baptista, P. M. (2018). Naturally-derived biomaterials for tissue engineering applications. In *Advances in Experimental Medicine and Biology* (Vol. 1077, pp. 421–449). https://doi.org/10.1007/978-981-13-0947-2_23.

Chen, A. A., Thomas, D. K., Ong, L. L., Schwartz, R. E., Golub, T. R., & Bhatia, S. N. (2011). Humanized mice with ectopic artificial liver tissues. *Proceedings of the National Academy of Sciences of the United States of America*, *108*(29), 11842–11847. https://doi.org/10.1073/pnas.1101791108.

Cui, H., Nowicki, M., Fisher, J. P., & Zhang, L. G. (2017). 3D Bioprinting for organ regeneration. *Advanced Healthcare Materials*, *6*(1), 1–29. https://doi.org/10.1002/adhm.201601118.

Dang, M., Saunders, L., Niu, X., Fan, Y., & Ma, P. X. (2018). Biomimetic delivery of signals for bone tissue engineering. In *Bone Research* (Vol. 6, Issue 1). https://doi.org/10.1038/s41413-018-0025-8.

Das, S., Pati, F., Choi, Y. J., Rijal, G., Shim, J. H., Kim, S. W., Ray, A. R., Cho, D. W., & Ghosh, S. (2015). Bioprintable, cell-laden silk fibroin-gelatin hydrogel supporting multilineage differentiation of stem cells for fabrication of three-dimensional tissue constructs. *Acta Biomaterialia*, *11*(1), 233–246. https://doi.org/10.1016/j.actbio.2014.09.023.

Fahy, N., Alini, M., & Stoddart, M. J. (2018). Mechanical stimulation of mesenchymal stem cells: Implications for cartilage tissue engineering. In *Journal of Orthopaedic Research* (Vol. 36, Issue 1). https://doi.org/10.1002/jor.23670.

Faulkner-Jones, A., Greenhough, S., A King, J., Gardner, J., Courtney, A., & Shu, W. (2013). Development of a valve-based cell printer for the formation of human embryonic stem cell spheroid aggregates. *Biofabrication*, *5*(1). https://doi.org/10.1088/1758-5082/5/1/015013.

Huh, D., Matthews, B. D., Mammoto, A., Montoya-Zavala, M., Yuan Hsin, H., & Ingber, D. E. (2010). Reconstituting organ-level lung functions on a chip. *Science*, *328*(5986), 1662–1668. https://doi.org/10.1126/science.1188302.

Jaramillo, M., Yeh, H., Yarmush, M. L., & Uygun, B. E. (2018). Decellularized human liver extracellular matrix (hDLM)-mediated hepatic differentiation of human induced pluripotent stem cells (hIPSCs). *Journal of Tissue Engineering and Regenerative Medicine*, *12*(4), e1962–e1973. https://doi.org/10.1002/term.2627.

Jia, W., Gungor-Ozkerim, P. S., Zhang, Y. S., Yue, K., Zhu, K., Liu, W., Pi, Q., Byambaa, B., Dokmeci, M. R., Shin, S. R., & Khademhosseini, A. (2016). Direct 3D bioprinting of perfusable vascular constructs using a blend bioink. *Biomaterials*, *106*, 58–68. https://doi.org/10.1016/j.biomaterials.2016.07.038.

Jorgensen, A. M., Yoo, J. J., & Atala, A. (2020). Solid organ bioprinting: strategies to achieve organ function. *Chemical Reviews*, *120*(19), 11093–11127. https://doi.org/10.1021/acs.chemrev.0c00145.

Kadota, Y., Yagi, H., Inomata, K., Matsubara, K., Hibi, T., Abe, Y., Kitago, M., Shinoda, M., Obara, H., Itano, O., & Kitagawa, Y. (2014). Mesenchymal stem cells support hepatocyte function in engineered liver grafts. *Organogenesis*, *10*(2), 268–277. https://doi.org/10.4161/org.27879.

Kakabadze, Z., Kakabadze, A., Chakhunashvili, D., Karalashvili, L., Berishvili, E., Sharma, Y., & Gupta, S. (2018). Decellularized human placenta supports hepatic tissue and allows rescue in acute liver failure. *Hepatology*, *67*(5), 1956–1969. https://doi.org/10.1002/hep.29713.

Kim, S. S., Utsunomiya, H., Koski, J. A., Wu, B. M., Cima, M. J., Sohn, J., Mukai, K., Griffith, L. G., & Vacanti, J. P. (1998). Survival and function of hepatocytes on a novel three-dimensional synthetic biodegradable polymer scaffold with an intrinsic network of channels. *Annals of Surgery*, *228*(1), 8–13. https://doi.org/10.1097/00000658-199807000-00002.

Kim, Y., Kang, K., Jeong, J., Paik, S. S., Kim, J. S., Park, S. A., Kim, W. D., Park, J., & Choi, D. (2017). Three-dimensional (3D) printing of mouse primary hepatocytes to generate 3D hepatic structure. *Annals of Surgical Treatment and Research*, *92*(2), 67–72. https://doi.org/10.4174/astr.2017.92.2.67.

Kizawa, H., Nagao, E., Shimamura, M., Zhang, G., & Torii, H. (2017). Scaffold-free 3D bio-printed human liver tissue stably maintains metabolic functions useful for drug discovery. *Biochemistry and Biophysics Reports*, *10*, 186–191. https://doi.org/10.1016/j.bbrep.2017.04.004.

Klein, S. G., Serchi, T., Hoffmann, L., Blömeke, B., & Gutleb, A. C. (2013). An improved 3D tetraculture system mimicking the cellular organisation at the alveolar barrier to study the potential toxic effects of particles on the lung. *Particle and Fibre Toxicology*, *10*(1), 1–17. https://doi.org/10.1186/1743-8977-10-31.

Ko, I. K., Peng, L., Peloso, A., Smith, C. J., Dhal, A., Deegan, D. B., Zimmerman, C., Clouse, C., Zhao, W., Shupe, T. D., Soker, S., Yoo, J. J., & Atala, A. (2015). Bioengineered transplantable porcine livers with re-endothelialized vasculature. *Biomaterials*, *40*, 72–79. https://doi.org/10.1016/j.biomaterials.2014.11.027.

Little, M. H., & Combes, A. N. (2019). Kidney organoids: Accurate models or fortunate accidents. *Genes and Development*, *33*(19–20), 1319–1345. https://doi.org/10.1101/gad.329573.119.

LoPresti, S. T., & Brown, B. N. (2018). Effect of source animal age upon macrophage response to extracellular matrix biomaterials. *Journal of Immunology and Regenerative Medicine*, *1*, 57–66. https://doi.org/10.1016/j.regen.2018.03.004

Neubauer, V. J., Döbl, A., & Scheibel, T. (2021). Silk-based materials for hard tissue engineering. *Materials*, *14*(3), 1–30. https://doi.org/10.3390/ma14030674.

Ong, C. S., Fukunishi, T., Zhang, H., Huang, C. Y., Nashed, A., Blazeski, A., Disilvestre, D., Vricella, L., Conte, J., Tung, L., Tomaselli, G. F., & Hibino, N. (2017). biomaterial-free three-dimensional bioprinting of cardiac tissue using human induced pluripotent stem cell derived cardiomyocytes. *Scientific Reports*, *7*(1), 1–11. https://doi.org/10.1038/s41598-017-05018-4.

Pagliuca, F. W., Millman, J. R., Gürtler, M., Segel, M., van Dervort, A., Ryu, J. H., Peterson, Q. P., Greiner, D., & Melton, D. A. (2014). Generation of functional human pancreatic β cells in vitro. *Cell*, *159*(2), 428–439. https://doi.org/10.1016/j.cell.2014.09.040.

Peneda Pacheco, D., Suárez Vargas, N., Visentin, S., & Petrini, P. (2021). From tissue engineering to engineering tissues: The role and application of: The vitro models. *Biomaterials Science*, *9*(1), 70–83. https://doi.org/10.1039/d0bm01097a.

Phillippi, J. A., Miller, E., Weiss, L., Huard, J., Waggoner, A., & Campbell, P. (2008). Microenvironments engineered by inkjet bioprinting spatially direct adult stem cells toward muscle- and bone-like subpopulations. *Stem Cells*, *26*(1). https://doi.org/10.1634/stemcells.2007-0520.

Rouwkema, J., Rivron, N. C., & van Blitterswijk, C. A. (2008). Vascularization in tissue engineering. *Trends in Biotechnology*, *26*(8), 434–441. https://doi.org/10.1016/j.tibtech.2008.04.009.

Rudolph, A. S. (1994). Biomaterial biotechnology using self-assembled lipid microstructures. *Journal of Cellular Biochemistry*, *56*(2), 183–187. https://doi.org/10.1002/jcb.240560211.

Salazar-Noratto, G. E., Luo, G., Denoeud, C., Padrona, M., Moya, A., Bensidhoum, M., Bizios, R., Potier, E., Logeart-Avramoglou, D., & Petite, H. (2020). Understanding and leveraging cell metabolism to enhance mesenchymal stem cell transplantation survival in tissue engineering and regenerative medicine applications. *Stem Cells*, *38*(1), 22–33. https://doi.org/10.1002/stem.3079.

Schubert, C., van Langeveld, M. C., & Donoso, L. A. (2014). Innovations in 3D printing: A 3D overview from optics to organs. *British Journal of Ophthalmology*, *98*(2), 159–161. https://doi.org/10.1136/bjophthalmol-2013-304446.

Stegemann, J. P., Kaszuba, S. N., & Rowe, S. L. (2007). Review: Advances in vascular tissue engineering using protein-based biomaterials. *Tissue Engineering*, *13*(11), 2601–2613. https://doi.org/10.1089/ten.2007.0196.

Stevens, K. R., Scull, M. A., Ramanan, V., Fortin, C. L., Chaturvedi, R. R., Knouse, K. A., Xiao, J. W., Fung, C., Mirabella, T., Chen, A. X., McCue, M. G., Yang, M. T., Fleming, H. E., Chung, K., de Jong, Y. P., Chen, C. S., Rice, C. M., & Bhatia, S. N. (2017). In situ expansion of engineered human liver tissue in a mouse model of chronic liver disease. *Science Translational Medicine*, *9*(399), 1–10. https://doi.org/10.1126/scitranslmed.aah5505.

Stevens, K. R., Ungrin, M. D., Schwartz, R. E., Ng, S., Carvalho, B., Christine, K. S., Chaturvedi, R. R., Li, C. Y., Zandstra, P. W., Chen, C. S., & Bhatia, S. N. (2013). InVERT molding for scalable control of tissue microarchitecture. *Nature Communications*, *4*, 1–11. https://doi.org/10.1038/ncomms2853.

Stupp, S. I. (2010). Self-assembly and biomaterials. *Nano Letters*, *10*(12), 4783–4786. https://doi.org/10.1021/nl103567y.

Tsang, V. L., Chen, A. A., Cho, L. M., Jadin, K. D., Sah, R. L., DeLong, S., West, J. L., & Bhatia, S. N. (2007). Fabrication of 3D hepatic tissues by additive photopatterning of cellular hydrogels. *The FASEB Journal*, *21*(3), 790–801. https://doi.org/10.1096/fj.06-7117com.

Underhill, G. H., Chen, A. A., Albrecht, D. R., & Bhatia, S. N. (2007). Assessment of hepatocellular function within PEG hydrogels. *Biomaterials*, *28*(2), 256–270. https://doi.org/10.1016/j.biomaterials.2006.08.043.

Zhang, X., Xie, Y., Koh, C. G., & Lee, L. J. (2009). A novel 3-D model for cell culture and tissue engineering. *Biomedical Microdevices*, *11*(4), 795–799. https://doi.org/10.1007/s10544-009-9294-8.

Chapter 12

In Vivo Applications of Bioprinting

Buket Er Urgancı*
Department of Medical Biology,
University of Pamukkale, Denizli, Turkey

Abstract

3D bioprinting is the most widely used method in tissue engineering and regenerative medicine. 3D bioprinting is an evolving technology with various applications in the construction of tissue and organ structures. Cells, growth factors, and biomaterials are combined to produce artificial tissues and organs to replace injured or diseased tissues and organs using 3D printing techniques. Biofunctional inks are the key component of 3D printing. It is relevant to select the right bioink by examining the typical properties of the organ and tissue produced and the printing technique. Selecting the biofunctional ink with suitable properties among different types of biofunctional inks increases the chance of success of the printed product. 3D microenvironments are created by 3D cell printing of in vivo tissues that mimic cellular activities like differentiation, proliferation, cell viability, and migration. However, more complex and astuter bioinks and more investigation are required to heal multicellular tissues and organs.

Keywords: 3D bioprinting, bioinks, in vivo application, tissue engineering

---

* Corresponding Author's Email: aber@pau.edu.tr.

In: Bioprinting the Human
Editors: Soner Şahin and Kenan Demir
ISBN: 978-1-68507-993-2

Introduction

In 3D printing technology, the desired textures are produced with three main fabrication strategies: inkjet bioprinting, microextrusion bioprinting, and laser-assisted bioprinting. Intercalarily, using multihead deposition systems (MHDS) allows multiple materials to be printed simultaneously or later.

Each technique has advantages and disadvantages over each other. Inkjet bioprinting, the oldest printing method, is based on the noncontact deposition of biofunctional ink droplets. This printing technique is preferred because of its compatibility with cells and materials, high printing speed, high cell viability, and low cost; however, it limits the use of high-viscosity materials.

Microextrusion bioprinting technology relies on pressing the ink by mechanical or pneumatic force, such as gas or pressure. This method provides the advantage of being able to print with high cell density and being compatible with high-viscosity materials. Although it provides low cost and easy compression, the pressure increased as the viscosity decreases negatively affects cell viability.

In laser-assisted bioprinting, cells are printed with a laser beam that vibrates at controlled speeds. Unlike the inkjet printing method, materials with a wide viscosity range can be printed with this method. In addition, since there is no spray system in laser-assisted printing, problems such as nozzle clogging are not encountered when compared to other techniques. However, it is quite expensive and requires a high gelation rate for high resolution.

Bioprinting Materials

In its most recent definition, biofabrication is the automated production of bioactive molecules, biomaterials, living cells, and cell clusters by bioprinting of micro-tissuesor and hybrid cell material structures, followed by the production of biofunctional products including the tissue maturation process.

The component that contains proteins, growth factors, cells, and/or biomolecules that are compatible with the physiological environment and are required for cell proliferation/differentiation is called bioink. They contain a biopolymer that acts as a 3D molecular scaffold from cells and which will enable these cells to develop and reproduce. It is this biopolymer gel that allows cells to be brought together to form tissues and printed on a 3D printer.

Amongst the most crucial factors for successful 3D bioprinting is the selection of appropriate biofunctional ink. In an ideal bioink, biological properties, material properties, many physical and mechanical properties should be present; These properties affect the printing time of the printed product, the morphological structure and durability of the printed material, the surface area and surface properties of the product, cell growth or differentiation, tissue viability, tissue healing, degradation time and biocompatibility (Camacho et al., 2019). Biocompatible bioinks to be used in 3D printing should ideally mimic the extracellular matrix (ECM) of the target tissue to support differentiation and cell proliferation. Since the spatial and temporal composition of the ECM changes during cell proliferation and differentiation, bioconnections should also reflect this dynamic evolution (Ostrovidov et al., 2019). Flow and fluency in the printing of bioink, that is, its rheological properties, are essential; low viscosity bioinks are adapted for inkjet bioprinting, while more viscous bioinks are generally preferred in extrusion bioprinting (Murphy et al., 2013). The viscosity and gelation time of the bioinkin are important for the solubility of the bioprinted structure and the preservation of its shape after printing. However, biolinks with high polymer concentration can be easily printed; They are generally unsuitable for cells, as they limit cell proliferation, migration, proliferation, and matrix remodeling (Holzl et al., 2016).

The hydrophilic nature of the selected ink and its surface properties also affect the role and success of the printed product in cell growth when applied to a living thing. Biofunctional inks have many biological properties such as oxygen exchange, toxic properties, and effect on cell regeneration. Choosing a synthetic or natural biofunctional ink has a direct effect on biological properties.

There is a trend towards the use of concentration (Colosi et al., 2016). In addition, a biolinker should ensure that cells are homogeneously dispersed in suspension to prevent cell aggregation and aggregation and to make larger structures, prolonging the time of bioprinting. The mechanical, chemical and morphological properties of the 3D printed structure should be similar to the targeted tissue. In addition, an environment should be created to protect cells from negative effects such as high temperature, organic solvents, and cross-linking agents during bioprinting. Printability, stability, biocompatibility, degradation time, nonbiological response, and viscosity are the main features to be considered in the selection of an ideal biofunctional ink.

The development of bioinks is an active area of research. Whether it contains bioink cells or not, it must be biocompatible. For this reason, the materials used in the bioink composition should not have a toxic effect even during the processes to be applied after 3D bioprinting, should have physicochemical properties such as viscosity required to produce 3D objects, and all of these properties, individually or together, should provide a suitable environment for cell viability. Sterile printing conditions must be met to obtain sufficient printing resolution for an accurate cell matrix structure while optimizing cell viability. In fact, the materials used in 3D bioprinting must be extruded, cross-linked, and biocompatible.

They must support growth and differentiation and maintain their shape for a period under various environmental conditions. The manufacturing process must be balanced between the requirements to produce robust biopolymer structures and achieve biologically relevant cell densities.

In various bioprinting strategies, biolinks are the fundamental component. They are settled or cross-linked during or immediately after bioprinting to form the last appearance of the intended tissue structures. The choice of biolinker is highly dependent on the specific implementation and cell type and also on the bioprinter to be used (Hong et al., 2017).

An ideal biobond should have desirable mechanical, biological, and chemical properties. These features should provide; i. Formation of structures with sufficient rigidity and mechanical strength while preserving tissue similarity ii. adjustable gelling and stabilization to aid in the bioprinting of highly conformable structures, iii. mimics the natural microenvironment, considering the biological similarity of tissues. iv. adequacy of chemical modifications to gather tissue-specific needs; and v. Large-scale production potential from small batches to multiple variants production (Loo et al., 2015). Determining the correct bioink formulation is the most important step for successful bioprinting. Various natural and synthetic biomaterials with certain traits have been used as bioinks to date. (Table 1).

Table 1. Different types of polymeric biofunctional inks

Protein based Bioinks	Collagen
	Gelatine
	Fibrinogen
Polysaccharide based	Alginate
	Gellan gum
	Hyaluronic acid
	Dextran
	Agarose
	Chitosan
Synthetic polymers	Polyethylene glycol
	Pluronic

Tissue Engineering

The traditional transplant approach cannot meet the increasing requirements for tissue/organ replacement. Tissue engineering is an alternative solution to organ shortage in organ transplantation. The purpose of bioprinting is to synthesize suitable tissues/organs de novo for the complete restoration of deteriorated, injured, or lost organs. (Wang et al., 2015).

3D printers are used in many fields, along with regenerative medicine and tissue engineering. 3D printers are also very important to meet the increasing need for organ transplantation worldwide. Of the 3D printing technique, biomimicry, self-assembly, or creating small tissue blocks are generally used. In recent studies, these methods have been developed and used to produce existing 3D human tissues and organs with mechanical and biological traits that are suitable for tissue and organ function (Hacioglu et al., 2018).

With bioprinting technology, bioactive molecules, cells, biomaterials, or cell clusters are printed to produce a structure. With this technology, it is aimed to mimic tissues and organs by developing the desired complex structures. Since the porosity, permeability, and mechanical properties of the printed structures can be adjusted, it makes it possible to design personalized functional tissues with computer-aided programs (Mobaraki et al., 2020).

In this application, biomaterials, cells, and other bioactive molecules are placed layer by layer to form delicate and complex structures that mimic tissues. Depending on the nature of the application, cells, bioactive molecules, and biomaterials can be imprinted together or separately, and thus they can undertake two separate tasks as both the imprint product and the tissue engineering scaffold (Murphy and Atara, 2014; Nakamura et al., 2010).

Tissue engineering is an interdisciplinary field of study in which engineering principles are applied to life sciences for tissue regeneration, regulation, and maintenance of organ functions (Lanza et al., 2020). The tissue engineering approach is based on the principle of producing living cells on in vitro biomaterial support scaffolds and placing the resulting cell-biomaterial structure in the damaged area in the body. In tissue engineering studies, the main goal in the long term is to create three-dimensional functional artificial tissues and organs using cells, tissue scaffolds and stimulating/regulatory factors instead of damaged organs that have become unable to function (O'brien, 2011). Three-dimensional (3D) bioprinting is the process of printing three-dimensional tissue in a biocompatible material, using a successive layer approach to create tissue structures in three-dimensional form, preserving cell function and viability (Murphy and Atala, 2014).

Studies continue on the creation of structures such as liver, kidney, blood vessels, and skin grafts with the three-dimensional bioprinting method (Kolesky et al., 2012). In tissue structures produced by bioprinting, strict control of external factors should be ensured in order for the cells to be viable and a precursor to tissue differentiation. Maintaining the integrity of the hydrogel, oxygen transfer, and medium continuity are important parameters. With this method, related cells can be isolated from tissue samples taken from the person by biopsy and produced in the desired amount and form by in vitro cultivation, and the immune response between the donor and the recipient in organ transplantation will be eliminated (Billet et al., 2012). This method, which is used in tissue engineering applications, skin grafts, cellular therapy, and drug release systems, also allows the physical behavior of cells to be examined in a three-dimensional environment such as in vivo (Auger et al., 2004).

The most important disadvantages of scaffolds obtained by conventional tissue engineering techniques are the pore size, porosity, and heterogeneity of interpore connections and scaffold geometry. In addition, cell-cell and cell-scaffold interactions are studied at the microenvironmental level. In order to achieve homogeneous cell distribution and seeding the desired number of cells, pipetting should not be done on the scaffold. The inability of cells to be placed in specific locations makes it nearly impossible to cultivate various cell types in specific patterns. It is known that various cell types do not settle randomly; on the contrary, they form a specific order according to their needs and functions in organs. For example, osteoblasts aggregate to form mineralized structures, while endothelial cells coalesce to form vessels. Therefore, a controlled positioning of cells on the scaffold is needed. The three-dimensional bioprinting method provides great advantages among other tissue engineering methods in terms of printing hydrogels and hybrid hydrogels with different and wide varieties of cells with high precision and resolution, production of complex geometries, and even printing of personalized products (Skardal et al., 2010).

Bone Tissue

Bone tissue is the most common type of hard tissue investigated in 3D bioprinting. The main challenge in this area is the fabrication of bone tissue structures with mechanical strength (Ahn et al., 2014). The structure of bone tissue must be porous for vascularization and cell proliferation (Bose et al.,2013). Biopolymer hybrid structures were constructed to use cell-loaded solutions to provide structural integrity and strength to bone tissue (Shim et al., 2012).

A structure for bone tissue regeneration was produced by printing amniotic fluid-derived stem (AFS) cells layer by layer on the HP Deskjet 550 printer with a bioink containing alginate and collagen. For in vivo assessment, the form was cultured in osteogenic medium for one week and subcutaneously implanted in nude mice. Densely packed hard bone-like material was constructed from mouse femur bone after 18 weeks (De Coppi et al., 2007).

Many attempts have been made to produce an osteochondral structure for tissue regeneration in areas of joint such as the knee. A group has produced a system that can print multiple biomaterials in an individual system. One was used to print a mixture of chondrocyte / alginate for cartilage growth, while others used the MG63 osteoblast cell line to create bone. The bioinks mentioned above were printed on polycaprolactone frames without a significant reduction in cell viability (Shim et al., 2012).

Various tissue forms of clinically useful proportion and completeness produced by a different research group with an integrated tissue-organ printer (ITOP) which was introduced to create multiple structures via a multicartridge module with a pneumatic extrusion system. This group formed the mandible and calvarial bone with a high cell viability of 91% and a high cell density of 5 x 106 cells/ml. The microchannels provided diffusion of oxygen and nutrients for cell proliferation even when the size of the construct was above the diffusion limit. Evaluation after 5 months of in vivo implantation of calvarial bone structures in mice, they observed a newly formed vascular network, which was considered a favorable sign for its ability to work in this clinical use. (Kang et al., 2016).

Skin Tissue

Skin is a complicated tissue composed of many different types of cell and functional structures, such as blood vessels, sweat glands, and hair follicles. Several 3D bioprinting research has been done in vitro and in vivo to create skin tissue, and skin healing has been successfully achieved. However, its thickness is limited due to the lack of vascularization that provides essential nutrients and oxygen to the cells. In addition, patient morbidity, low dependence on the surrounding natural texture, and high cost of production are some of the restrictions that need to be resolved.

Another group studied in vivo bioprinting of skin tissues using mesenchymal stem cells (MSC) or amniotic fluid-derived stem cells (AFS), which were suspended in fibrin/collagen gels to bioprint on the skin wound of a nude mouse for the recovery of a large wound in a mouse model (Skardal et al. 2012).

Keratinocyte/collagen layers and fibroblast/collagen layers on a Matriderm film printed, and they coated skin wounds using dorsal skin folds of nude mice. The construct was completely attached to the surrounding tissue and keratinocytes formed a dense, multilayered epidermis after 11 days. Additionally, some blood vessels were observed growing from wound beds and edges toward printed cells (Michael et al., 2013).

The electrosprayed skin tissue construct was subcutaneously implanted on the dorsal side of the mice, showing that bioelectrospraying did not significantly affect cell viability and functionality. Two days after implantation, no damage was observed in the cells by H&E staining (Jayasinghe et al., 2011).

Other Tissues

Many studies have been related to the use of bioprinting for skin and bone regeneration. The efficiency of printing the cell-suspended biomaterial on a desired architecture is directly proportional to the creation of artificial vascular structures. Difficulties in mimicking the biological and mechanical properties of blood vessels make bioprinting difficult to perform experimentally (Hoch et al., 2014).

Post-imprint differentiation can be added to the bioprinting process of tissue or organ to differentiate printed cells into desired cell types. With this technique, a miniliver was generated from both human induced pluripotent stem cells (hiPSCs) and maturing human embryonic stem cells (hESCs) to be hepatocyte-like cells. The group created a 3D alginate matrix and constructed the structure using a valve-based bioprinting system that did not adversely affect cell viability. An examination carried out after a 21-day specialization protocol proved that the structure was hepatic with peak albumin secretion. (Faulkner-Jones et al., 2015).

Neural cells have regenerative and neuroprotective potential. It allows for the replenishment of unfunctional or impaired neural tissues by locating neural stem cells in the appropriate zone. With a 3D bioprinting system, it can preserve cell-to-cell communication, which is an important feature of nervous tissue and can be achieved with the morphological structure, by creating highly controlled geometries of biomaterials in neural tissue development (Zhu et al., 2014).

Conclusion

3D microenvironments are created by 3D cell printing of bioinks in vivo tissues that mimic cellular activities such as migration, cell viability, differentiation, and proliferation. However, more research is needed to solve the vascularization problem. In addition, more complex and astuter bioinks and more research are required to heal multicellular tissues and organs.

Printing large sizes of tissues and organs requires a long production time. Storage of cell biomaterial suspensions for a long time is the major limitation of epitomizing living cells in biomaterials. This restriction limits cell bioactivity and compromises its viability. Therefore, a more automated and faster way of loading and maintaining the cell biomaterial suspension for tissue and organ production is required.

References

Ahn, S., Lee, H., Lee, E. J., Kim, G. (2014). A direct cell printing supplemented with low-temperature processing method for obtaining highly porous three-dimensional cell-laden scaffolds. *Journal of Materials Chemistry*, 2(18):2773–2782.

Auger, F. A., Berthod, F., Moulin, V., Pouliot, R., Germain, L. (2004). Tissue-engineered skin substitutes: from in vitro constructs to in vivo applications. *Biotechnol Appl. Biochem.*, 39, 263-75.

Billiet, T., Vandenhaute, M., Schelfhout, J., Van Vlierberghe, S., Dubruel, P. (2012). A review of trends and limitations in hydrogel-rapid prototyping for tissue engineering. *Biomaterials,* 33, 6020-41.

Bose, S., Vahabzadeh, S., Bandyopadhyay, A. (2013). Bone tissue engineering using 3D printing. *Materials Today*, 16(12),496–504.

Camacho, P., Busari, H., Seims, K. B., Tolbert, J. W., Chow, L. W. (2019). Materials as bioinks and bioink design. In: Güvendiren, M. (Editors), *3D Bioprinting in Medicine Technologies, Bioinks, and Applications* (67-100), Springer, Switzerland.

Colosi, C., Shin, S. R., Manoharan, V., Massa, S., Costantini, M., Barbetta, A., Dokmeci, M. R., Dentini, M., Khademhosseini, A. (2016). Microfluidic bioprinting of heterogeneous 3D tissue constructs using low-viscosity bioink. *Adv. Mater.*, 28(4), 677-84.

De Coppi, P., Bartsch, G., Siddiqui, M. M., Xu, T., Santos, C. C., Perin, L., Mostoslavsky, G., Serre, A. C., Snyder, E. Y., Yoo, J. J. (2007). Isolation of amniotic stem cell lines with potential for therapy. *Nature Biotechnology*, 25(1), 100–106.

Faulkner-Jones, A., Fyfe, C., Cornelissen, D-J, Gardner, J., King, J., Courtney A, Shu W (2015). Bioprinting of human pluripotent stem cells and their directed differentiation into hepatocyte-like cells for the generation of mini-livers in 3D. *Biofabrication*, 7(4), 044102

Hacıoğlu, A., Yılmazer, H., Ustundag, C.B. (2018). 3D Printing for tissue engineering applications. *Journal of Polytechnic*, 21, 1, 221-227.

Hoch, E., Tovar, G. E., Borchers, K. (2014). Bioprinting of artificial blood vessels: current approaches towards a demanding goal. *European Journal of Cardio-Thoracic Surgery*, 46(5), 767– 778.

Hölzl, K., Lin, S., Tytgat, L., Van Vlierberghe, S., Gu, L., Ovsianikov, A. (2016). Bioink properties before, during and after 3D bioprinting. *Biofabrication*, 8(3), 032002.

Hong, N., Yang, G. H., Lee, J., Kim, G. (2018). 3D bioprinting and its in vivo applications. *J. Biomed. Mater. Res. B Appl. Biomater.*, 106(1), 444-459.

Jayasinghe, S. N., Warnes, G., Scotton, C. J. (2011). Bio-electrosprayed Living Composite Matrix Implanted into Mouse Models. *Macromolecular Bioscience*, 11(10), 1364–1369. 2011

Kang, H-W., Lee, S. J., Ko, I. K., Kengla, C., Yoo, J. J., Atala, A. (2016). A 3D bioprinting system to produce human-scale tissue constructs with structural integrity. *Nature Biotechnology*, 34(3), 312–319.

Kolesky, D. B., Truby, R. L., Gladman, A., Busbee, T. A., Homan, K. A., Lewis, J. A. (2014). 3D bioprinting of vascularized, heterogeneous cell-laden tissue constructs. *Adv. Mater.*, 26, 3124-30.

Lanza, R., Langer, R., Vacanti, J. P. (2020). *Principles of Tissue Engineering*. Academic Press.

Loo, Y., Lakshmanan, A., Ni, M., Toh, L. L., Wang, S., Hauser, C. A. (2015). Peptide Bioink: Self-assembling nanofibrous scaffolds for three-dimensional organotypic cultures. *Nano Lett.*, 15(10), 6919-25.

Michael, S., Sorg, H., Peck, C-T., Koch, L., Deiwick, A., Chichkov, B., Vogt, P. M., Reimers, K. (2013). Tissue engineered skin substitutes created by laser-assisted bioprinting form skin-like structures in the dorsal skin fold chamber in mice. *PloS One*, 8(3), e57741.

Mobaraki, M., Ghaffari, M., Yazdanpanah, A., Luo, Y., Mills, D.K. (2020) Bioinks and bioprinting: A focused review. *Bioprinting*, 18, e00080.

Murphy, S. V., Atala, A. (2014). 3D bioprinting of tissues and organs. *Nature Biotechnology*, 32(8), 773.

Murphy, S. V., Skardal, A., Atala, A. (2013). Evaluation of hydrogels for bio-printing applications. *J. Biomed. Mater. Res.*, 101A, 272–284.

Nakamura, M., Iwanaga, S., Henmi, C., Arai, K., Nishiyama, Y. (2010). Biomatrices and biomaterials for future developments of bioprinting and biofabrication. *Biofabrication*, 2(1), 014110.

O'Brien, F. J. (2011). Biomaterials & scaffolds for tissue engineering. *Mater. Today*, 14, 88-95.

Ostrovidov, S., Salehi, S., Costantini, M., Suthiwanich, K., Ebrahimi, M., Sadeghian, R. B. and et al., (2019). 3D bioprinting in skeletal muscle tissue engineering. *Small*, 15, 1805530.

Shim, J-H., Lee, J-S., Kim, J. Y., Cho, D-W. (2012). Bioprinting of a mechanically enhanced three-dimensional dual cell-laden construct for osteochondral tissue engineering using a multi-head tissue/organ building system. *Journal of Micromechanics and Microengineering*, 22(8), 085014.

Skardal, A., Mack, D., Kapetanovic, E., Atala, A., Jackson, J. D., Yoo, J., Soker, S. (2012). Bioprinted amniotic fluid-derived stem cells accelerate healing of large skin wounds. *Stem Cells Translational Medicine*, 1(11), 792–802.

Skardal, A., Zhang, J., Prestwich, G. D. (2010). Bioprinting vessel-like constructs using hyaluronan hydrogels crosslinked with tetrahedral polyethylene glycol tetra crylates. *Biomaterials*, 31, 6173-81.

Wang, M. Y., He, J. K., Liu, Y. X., et al., (2015). The trend towards in vivo bioprinting. *International Journal of Bioprinting*, 1(1), 15–26.

Zhu, W., O'Brien, C., O'Brien, J. R., Zhang, L. G. (2014). 3D nano/microfabrication techniques and nanobiomaterials for neural tissue regeneration. *Nanomedicine*, 9(6), 859– 875.

Chapter 13

3D Bioprinting in Cancer Research

Mücahit Seçme*
Department of Medical Biology, Faculty of Medicine,
Pamukkale University, Denizli, Turkey

Abstract

Bioprinting offers the opportunity to create complex 3D architectural structures for living cell systems. Bioprinting technology has gained considerable popularity and applicability in many research fields such as bioengineering and medicine. Bioprinting enables more effective and rapid modeling and usages of macromolecules, cellular systems, and biological materials. Recent developments in this technology provide great potential for research and application studies in the field of cancer. Bioprinted 3D cancer models provide a more comprehensive and complex modelling opportunity, providing cell-cell, cell-matrix interactions and a wider range of physiological, biological, and structural study opportunities. 3D cancer bioprinting research contributes to understanding the pathophysiology of cancer and the development of anticancer agents, making models that mimic the tumor micro-environment, and thus contributing to cancer diagnosis and treatment studies.

Keywords: 3D bioprinting, cancer models, tumorigenesis

---

* Corresponding Author's Email: mehtersecme@gmail.com.

In: Bioprinting the Human
Editors: Soner Şahin and Kenan Demir
ISBN: 978-1-68507-993-2

Introduction

Cancer is one of the leading causes of death worldwide, with approximately 19.3 million new cases and 9.9 million cancer-related deaths in 2020, and is one of the deadly diseases that affect the whole world (Sung et al., 2021). In general, the cancer incidence and mortality burden are increasing rapidly all over the world. Cancer therapy is among the main research focus for the pharmacology industry, personalized medicine, and biomedical research (Liu et al., 2019; Sung et al., 2021). The existence of many cancer types and subtypes and the highly complex molecular biological structures of each of them complicate the treatment of the disease and require a rapid and effective treatment strategy (Palanisamy et al., 2010; Berer et al., 2011). To better understand cancer progression, 3D cancer models are needed that can closely mimic the *in vivo* tumor microenvironment and enable us to observe the complex mechanism of cancer and its pathophysiology. Given these challenges and needs, bioprinting offers the ability to create cancer tissue models for research and has the potential to significantly accelerate this research (Knowlton et al., 2015). Complex and three-dimensional *in vivo* tumor microenvironments are of great importance in cancer initiation and progression. Most *in vitro* cancer modelling studies use methods based on planar 2D geometry, which are far from being able to accurately mimic tumor initiation and progression. (Knowlton et al., 2015; Oztan et al., 2020).

Studies conducted to compare 2D and 3D cancer models have revealed differences between the two models in many cellular events ((Knowlton et al., 2015) such as protein (Ridky et al., 2010) and mRNA expression levels in cells (Ghosh et al., 2005), cell migration (Friedl and Wolf, 2010), responses to drugs (Loessner et al., 2010), signal transduction (Kim et al., 2013) cell morphology, viability, proliferation, and cell organization (Chopra et al., 1997; Li et al., 2008). Although 2D cultures provide important hypothetical results regarding cancer pathogenesis, it is necessary to evaluate cancer cells *in vivo*, especially considering cell-cell and cell-matrix interactions, in order to determine more physiologically holistic results at the organism level. Therefore, it can be thought that 3D models will provide more effective and accurate observation opportunities than 2D studies in terms of cancer microenvironment and biological behaviour (Knowlton et al., 2015).

3D printing is the process of making solid three-dimensional objects from computer-aided designs, a digital file, where lead materials are deposited layer by layer and additive manufacturing is used to create complex 3D geometries (Freedman, 2012; Al-Maliki and Al-Maliki, 2015). In the next period, 3D printing in biology and medicine has developed into the field of bioprinting, including cell applications, extracellular matrix, and biomaterials (Mironov et al., 2003; Xiang et al., 2022). Conventional printing methods, such as photolithography, soft lithography, and microstamping, have the advantage of creating geometrically complex scaffolds for living cells (Mironov et al., 2008). These advantages open up a wide variety of uses of bioprinting in areas such as basic cellular and oncological research, disease modelling, regenerative medicine, and pharmacology, including the design of 3D tissue structures (Knowlton et al., 2015). In this context, 3D bioprinting in cancer research allows the repositioning of the *in vivo* tumor microenvironment with high accuracy and contributes to the bioengineering technology in cancer research. In these studies, the aim is to allow the use of cells and biomaterials obtained from patients, develop drugs and effective agents that can be produced within the scope of personalized medicine, and increase the capacities of existing strategies in cancer modeling. In particular, bioprinted 3D cancer models are expected to fill the gap between classical cell culture and experimental animal studies, and can also replace animal models in research in the field of medicine, depending on developing technology and scientific advances (Zhang et al., 2016; Liu et al., 2019).

In relation to cancer biology, the complex tumor microenvironment and the interactions of cells of different origins in this environment with the environment and with each other constitute a heterogeneous structure. And this situation constitutes a hierarchical and holistic structure (Polyak et al., 2009). Existing cell culture working systems have not been able to fully model this complexity. It is believed that more effective working strategies can be developed by better imitating this complex structure and tumor microenvironment with 3D cell models. 3D bioprinting will provide the necessary biomaterials and the relationship between multiple cell types, extracellular matrix, and microenvironment, and enable easy experimental methods in a reproducible manner (Zhang et al., 2016; Charbe et al., 2017; Liu et al., 2019).

Applications of Bioprinted Cancer Models

Tumor Angiogenesis

Angiogenesis is one of the necessary steps for transport of nutrients and oxygen, which is an important requirement for cancer cells, and one of the most important difficulties in 3D cancer models is the insufficiency of this vascular network. (Jain et al., 2005). However, advances have been made in integrating the vascular network and cells with developments in bioprinting technology. For example, demonstrating that vascular endothelial cells can be made vascular in hydrogel matrices to mimic blood vessels has made it possible to model vascularization (Vivian et al., 2015; Liu et al., 2019). With the help of technologies such as microfluidic bioprinting and stereolithography, other bioprinting methods have also contributed to angiogenesis studies in cancer research (Jia et al., 2016; Pi et al., 2018; Miri et al., 2018).

Tumor Spheroid Formation

A study on the applications of 3D bioprinting strategies on spheroid structures has been demonstrated in breast cancer (Hribar et al., 2015). In the study with BT474 breast cancer cells, narrower sized spheroids were observed in 3D modelling compared to flat cell culture. It has also been shown that the expression of Hypoxia inducible factor-1 alpha (HIF-1α) is consistent in 3D cultured spheroids compared to previous tumor spheroids. It has shown that 3D bioprinting platforms can be useful in the context of low-cost effective outcome and accurate tumor modelling strategies of tumor progression, cell migration, colony formation, and other cancer steps (Hribar et al., 2015; Knowlton et al., 2015).

Tumor Microenvironment

In addition to cancer cells, there is a stroma composed of a large number and variety of untransformed cells, growth factors, cytokines, and a specialized extracellular matrix (ECM) in tumor tissue. Recent findings suggest that tumorigenesis is highly dependent on contextual signals from the tumor-associated microenvironment. Cancer-associated stroma provides continuous and active support to carcinoma cells through various pathophysiological processes that modulate tumor progression (Hanahan, and Weinberg, 2000; Bhowmick et al., 2004). Taking into account the tumor microenvironment as a whole in cancer research, it is important that the model to be emulated is a comprehensive structure that contains both the extracellular matrix, cancer-associated fibroblasts, and lymphocytes and other immune cells. In this context, 3D bioprinting platforms are believed to allow for more holistic research as they allow the creation of this complex structure (Liu et al., 2019). In a study, a brain model was created with the 3D bioprinting system, in which the dynamic interactions of both macrophages and glioblastoma cells were modelled (Heinrich et al., 2019).

Tumor Metastasis

It is thought that using 3D bioprinting systems will enable more reliable and sensitive studies to be carried out, especially for metastasis, which is one of the important steps of cancer, and will make a significant contribution to tumor studies (Lopes et al., 2017; Liu et al. .2019). In a study, an *in vitro* bone matrix was created using 3D bioprinting platforms. In this context, using a tabletop stereolithography-based 3D bioprinting technique, a biomimetic environment has been presented that will allow MDA-MB-231 breast cancer cells to metastasize. In addition, a model with both breast cancer cells and mesenchymal stem cells was designed and implemented in the printed 3D bone matrix in this way (Zhu et al., 2016).

Anticancer Drug Development and Therapeutic Screening

Immunosuppressive mice or genetically modified animal models, 2D cell culture studies are important tools in oncology research and enable many studies such as pharmacodynamics, pharmacokinetic toxicology, geno-toxicity, and gene expression changes (Charbe et al., 2017). 3D bioprinting systems provide a good platform to investigate the anticancer activities and therapeutic potentials of various agents in cancer modelling studies. The existence of 3D bioprinting systems is positively evaluated in achieving more promising results from the low successes experienced in the development of cancer drugs (May, 2018). 3D bioprinting models, efficacy, side effects, and coculture studies allow both normal and cancerous cells to be studied together. The fact that 3D bioprinting models can present a biomimetic model suggests that they can contribute to biological and physiological studies and observations more effectively than normal flat culture studies. In a study on doxorubicin and drug resistance, a 3D bioprinting model was created in the matrix in which mesenchymal stem cells derived from adipose tissue and

HER2 positive breast cancer cells were embedded, and successful results were obtained (Wang et al., 2018).

Conclusıon

3D bioprinting applications of tissue and organ models is an emerging research area that has gained a lot of importance recently. 3D bioprinting has many uses, especially oncology research, regenerative medicine, biomedical fields, drug discovery and effectiveness, and so on. Due to the development of 3D bioprinting techniques, it is now possible to work with realistic tissue, organ, and cellular cancer models. The realization of problems or difficulties in classical 2D cell culture and animal models with more reliable and effective 3D bioprinting studies will lead to many biomedical researches, especially oncology research. 3D bioprinting techniques also have the potential to change the process in phase studies and clinical trials after preclinical research. These newly developed 3D bioprinting applications, in addition to making clinical trials more effective, accelerate the discovery process of new drugs and agents ready for clinical use and reduce the economic cost in this area. In the following years, developments in 3D bioprinting models and the spread of their usage areas will replace 2D cell culture and animal models and thus will shed light on the more reliable evaluation of preclinical studies. Unique advances in 3D bioprinting technology can help overcome the existing challenges of complex organ and tissue engineering (Charbe et al., 2017).

Another promising potential for 3D bioprinting is the use of patients' own immune cells, stromal cells, or cancer cells, to implement a more effective treatment strategy, and, in this context, to contribute to the development of personalized medicine. Although *in vivo* cancer model studies with 3D bioprinting can fully mimic the tumor microenvironment and cell culture, the difficulties in combining different cell culture conditions can be overcome depending on the developing technology over time. In conclusion, 3D bioprinting has become an important platform for cancer model research, as it allows the development of anticancer agents and drugs, facilitates cancer treatment regimens and research within the scope of personalized medicine, and also facilitates the study of cancer biology and pathology (Liu et al., 2019).

References

Berger, M. F., Lawrence, M. S., Demichelis, F., Drier, Y., Cibulskis, K., et al., (2011). The genomic complexity of primary human prostate cancer. *Nature,* 470(7333), 214–220. https://doi.org/10.1038/nature09744.

Bhowmick, N. A., Neilson, E. G., & Moses, H. L. (2004). Stromal fibroblasts in cancer initiation and progression. *Nature,* 432(7015), 332–337. https://doi.org/10.1038/nature03096.

Charbe, N., McCarron, P. A., & Tambuwala, M. M. (2017). Three-dimensional bio-printing: A new frontier in oncology research. *World Journal of Clinical Oncology,* 8(1), 21–36. https://doi.org/10.5306/wjco.v8.i1.21.

Chopra, V., Dinh, T. V., & Hannigan, E. V. (1997). Three-dimensional endothelial-tumor epithelial cell interactions in human cervical cancers. *In Vitro Cellular & Developmental Biology Animal,* 33(6), 432–442. https://doi.org/10.1007/s11626-997-0061-y.

Freedman, D. H. (2012) Layer by layer. *Technol. Rev.* 115, 50–53.

Friedl, P., & Wolf, K. (2010). Plasticity of cell migration: a multiscale tuning model. *The Journal of Cell Biology,* 188(1), 11–19. https://doi.org/10.1083/jcb.200909003.

Ghosh, S., Spagnoli, G. C., Martin, I., Ploegert, S., Demougin, P., Heberer, M., & Reschner, A. (2005). Three-dimensional culture of melanoma cells profoundly affects gene expression profile: a high density oligonucleotide array study. *Journal of Cellular Physiology,* 204(2), 522–531. https://doi.org/10.1002/jcp.20320.

Hanahan, D., & Weinberg, R. A. (2000). The hallmarks of cancer. *Cell,* 100(1), 57–70. https://doi.org/10.1016/s0092-8674(00)81683-9.

Heinrich, M. A., Bansal, R., Lammers, T., Zhang, Y. S., Michel Schiffelers, R., & Prakash, J. (2019). 3D-bioprinted mini-brain: a glioblastoma model to study cellular interactions and therapeutics. *Advanced Materials (Deerfield Beach, Fla.),* 31(14), e1806590. https://doi.org/10.1002/adma.201806590.

Hribar, K. C., Finlay, D., Ma, X., Qu, X., Ondeck, M. G., Chung, P. H., Zanella, F., Engler, A. J., Sheikh, F., Vuori, K., & Chen, S. C. (2015). Nonlinear 3D projection printing of concave hydrogel microstructures for long-term multicellular spheroid and embryoid body culture. *Lab on a Chip,* 15(11), 2412–2418. https://doi.org/10.1039/c5lc00159e.

Jabbar Qasim Al-Maliki and Alaa Jabbar Qasim Al-Maliki, The processes and technologies of 3d printing. *International Journal of Advance in Computer Science and Technology.* 4 (10) (2015) 161-165.

Jain, R. K., Au, P., Tam, J., Duda, D. G., & Fukumura, D. (2005). Engineering vascularized tissue. *Nature Biotechnology,* 23(7), 821–823. https://doi.org/10.1038/nbt0705-821.

Jia W, Gungor-Ozkerim P. S., Zhang Y. S. et al. Direct 3D bioprinting of perfusable vascular constructs using a Blend Bioink. *Biomaterials* 106, 58–68 (2016).

Kim, B. J., Hannanta-anan, P., Chau, M., Kim, Y. S., Swartz, M. A., & Wu, M. (2013). Cooperative roles of SDF-1α and EGF gradients on tumor cell migration revealed by a robust 3D microfluidic model. *PloS one,* 8(7), e68422. https://doi.org/10.1371/journal.pone.0068422.

Knowlton, S., Onal, S., Yu, C. H., Zhao, J. J., & Tasoglu, S. (2015). Bioprinting for cancer research. *Trends in Biotechnology,* 33(9), 504–513. https://doi.org/10.1016/j.tibtech.2015.06.007.

Li, C. L., Tian, T., Nan, K. J., Zhao, N., Guo, Y. H., Cui, J., Wang, J., & Zhang, W. G. (2008). Survival advantages of multicellular spheroids vs. monolayers of HepG2 cells in vitro. *Oncology Reports,* 20(6), 1465–1471.

Liu, T., Delavaux, C., & Zhang, Y. S. (2019). 3D bioprinting for oncology applications. *Journal of 3D Printing in Medicine*, 3(2), 55–58. https://doi.org/10.2217/3dp-2019-0004.

Loessner, D., Stok, K. S., Lutolf, M. P., Hutmacher, D. W., Clements, J. A., & Rizzi, S. C. (2010). Bioengineered 3D platform to explore cell-ECM interactions and drug resistance of epithelial ovarian cancer cells. *Biomaterials,* 31(32), 8494–8506. https://doi.org/10.1016/j.biomaterials.2010.07.064.

López-Soto, A., Gonzalez, S., Smyth, M. J., & Galluzzi, L. (2017). Control of Metastasis by NK Cells. *Cancer Cell,* 32(2), 135–154. https://doi.org/10.1016/j.ccell.2017.06.009.

May M. (2018). Cancer research with a human touch. *Nature,* 556(7700), 259–261. https://doi.org/10.1038/d41586-018-04161-w.

Miri A, Nieto D, Iglesias L et al. Microfluidics-enabled multimaterial maskless stereolithographic bioprinting. *Adv. Mater.* 30(27), 1800242 (2018).

Mironov, V., Boland, T., Trusk, T., Forgacs, G., & Markwald, R. R. (2003). Organ printing: computer-aided jet-based 3D tissue engineering. *Trends in Biotechnology,* 21(4), 157–161. https://doi.org/10.1016/S0167-7799(03)00033-7.

Mironov, V., Kasyanov, V., Drake, C., & Markwald, R. R. (2008). Organ printing: promises and challenges. *Regenerative Medicine,* 3(1), 93–103. https://doi.org/10.2217/17460751.3.1.93.

Oztan, Y. C., Nawafleh, N., Zhou, Y., Liyanage, P. Y., Hettiarachchi, S. D., Seven, E. S., Leblanc, R. M., Ouhtit, A., & Celik, E. (2020). Recent advances on utilization of bioprinting for tumor modeling. *Bioprinting (Amsterdam, Netherlands),* 18, 10.1016/j.bprint.2020.e00079. https://doi.org/10.1016/j.bprint.2020.e00079.

Palanisamy, N., Ateeq, B., Kalyana-Sundaram, S., Pflueger, D., Ramnarayanan, K., Shankar, S., Han, B., Cao, Q., Cao, X., Suleman, K., Kumar-Sinha, C., Dhanasekaran, S. M., Chen, Y. B., Esgueva, R., Banerjee, S., LaFargue, C. J., Siddiqui, J., Demichelis, F., Moeller, P., Bismar, T. A., Chinnaiyan, A. M. (2010). Rearrangements of the RAF kinase pathway in prostate cancer, gastric cancer and melanoma. *Nature Medicine,* 16(7), 793–798. https://doi.org/10.1038/nm.2166.

Pi Q, Maharjan S, Yan X et al. Digitally tunable microfluidic bioprinting of multilayered cannular tissues. *Adv. Mater.* 30(43), 1706913 (2018).

Polyak, K., Haviv, I., & Campbell, I. G. (2009). Co-evolution of tumor cells and their microenvironment. *Trends in Genetics: TIG,* 25(1), 30–38. https://doi.org/10.1016/j.tig.2008.10.012.

Ridky, T. W., Chow, J. M., Wong, D. J., & Khavari, P. A. (2010). Invasive three-dimensional organotypic neoplasia from multiple normal human epithelia. *Nature Medicine,* 16(12), 1450–1455. https://doi.org/10.1038/nm.2265.

Sung, H., Ferlay, J., Siegel, R. L., Laversanne, M., Soerjomataram, I., Jemal, A., & Bray, F. (2021). Global Cancer Statistics 2020: GLOBOCAN Estimates of incidence and mortality worldwide for 36 cancers in 185 countries. *CA: A Cancer Journal for Clinicians*, 71(3), 209–249. https://doi.org/10.3322/caac.21660.

Vivian K. L., Vivian K. G. D., Vivian K. H. Z., Vivian K. S. S. Y. *Generation of 3-D Glioblastoma-Vascular Niche Using 3-D Bioprinting.* Presented at: 41st Annual Northeast Biomedical Engineering Conference, Boston, MA, USA, 17–19 April 2015.

Wang, Y., Shi, W., Kuss, M., Mirza, S., Qi, D., Krasnoslobodtsev, A., Zeng, J., Band, H., Band, V., & Duan, B. (2018). 3D Bioprinting of breast cancer models for drug resistance study. *ACS Biomaterials Science & Engineering,* 4(12), 4401–4411. https://doi.org/10.1021/acsbiomaterials.8b01277.

Xiang, Y., Miller, K., Guan, J., Kiratitanaporn, W., Tang, M., & Chen, S. (2022). 3D bioprinting of complex tissues in vitro: state-of-the-art and future perspectives. *Archives of Toxicology,* 96(3), 691–710. https://doi.org/10.1007/s00204-021-03212-y.

Zhang, Y. S., Duchamp, M., Oklu, R., Ellisen, L. W., Langer, R., & Khademhosseini, A. (2016). Bioprinting the Cancer Microenvironment. *ACS Biomaterials Science & Engineering,* 2(10), 1710–1721. https://doi.org/10.1021/acsbiomaterials.6b00246.

Zhu, W., Holmes, B., Glazer, R. I., & Zhang, L. G. (2016). 3D printed nanocomposite matrix for the study of breast cancer bone metastasis. *Nanomedicine: Nanotechnology, Biology, and Medicine,* 12(1), 69–79. https://doi.org/10.1016/j.nano.2015.09.010.

Editors' Contact Information

Dr. Soner Şahin, MD
Professor, Faculty of Medicine,
Department of Neurosurgery,
Nisantasi University, Istanbul, Turkey
sahin.soner@nisantasi.edu.tr

Dr. Kenan Demir, MD
Health Sciences University,
Samsun Training and Research Hospital,
İlkadım, Turkey
kenandemir@hotmail.com

Index

S

T

V